FOUR SEASONS FOR
Charlotte

by

RACHEL REYNOLDS

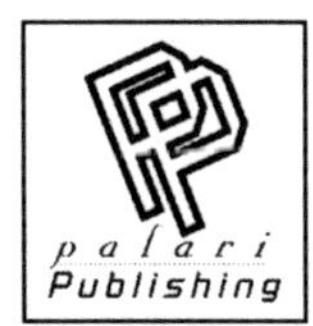

palari
Publishing

All photos are from the author's collection and permission has been obtained where required.

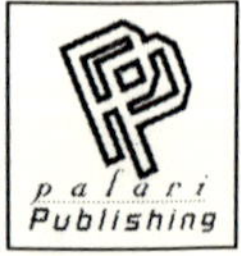 Publishing by Palari Publishing, LLP
Richmond, VA
www.PalariBooks.com

Library of Congress Cataloging-in-Publication Data: Applied for

ISBN 9781928662259

Cover design by Ted Randler
Cover photo by Jamie E. Tamm

Acknowledgements

This book has been a labor of love. Gratitude is due to many:

Thank you to CaringBridge for providing the early framework for our blog. It's because of your organization that we were able to share our story quickly and easily with the world.

To Bob and Meryl, thank you for the use of Shangri-Log as I finished the first draft of the manuscript.

To Phyllis and Lia, thank you for reading early drafts and providing editorial notes. Thank you also to Colleen and Dave for additional editorial guidance.

To Phyllis and Kate, thank you for guiding me as I navigated the world of publishing.

Thank you to my family for their unwavering support.

Thank you to *The Network* for their unending acts of kindness.

Thank you to everyone who said, "You should really write a book about this."

To Susan Greenbaum, Sting, Eddie From Ohio, Peter Gabriel, Nickel Creek, Bobby McFerrin, Vampire Weekend, Pomplamoose, Jonathan Coulton, and The Barenaked Ladies (among others) for providing musical inspiration while I wrote chapter after chapter.

Thank you to my mother, Gayellen. When I search for strength, you are one of my biggest inspirations. Thank you for always believing in your children and supporting them through any challenge life seems to bring.

A special thank you to Roger. This book is not just my story; it's our story. He read the early drafts and gave me words when writer's block had me stuck. More importantly, he makes me laugh when I want to cry. He remains my solid rock whenever life is stormy.

Finally, thank you to Charlotte. Thank you for coming into my life. Thank you for sharing your spirit for fifty-four short months. I am proud to be your mama.

Table of Contents

Acknowledgements 3

1   Do You Have Children? 7

2   The Day Our Lives Changed Forever 11

3   Hospital Time 25
      Lesson Learned #1 46

4   Course of Treatment 49

5   The New Normal 57

6   The Network 63
      Lesson Learned #2 71

7   Circles of Faith 73
      Lesson Learned #3 81

8   Timeline 83

9   What Are You In For? 91

10   Bringing up Baby… 97

11   On the Other Side of the Table 103
      Lesson Learned #4 109

12   It Can Always Get Worse 111

13   The Journey to the Terminal 117

14   Charlotte's Farewell Tour 123

15   What Can You Say? 137

Epilogue: Charlotte's Legacy 147

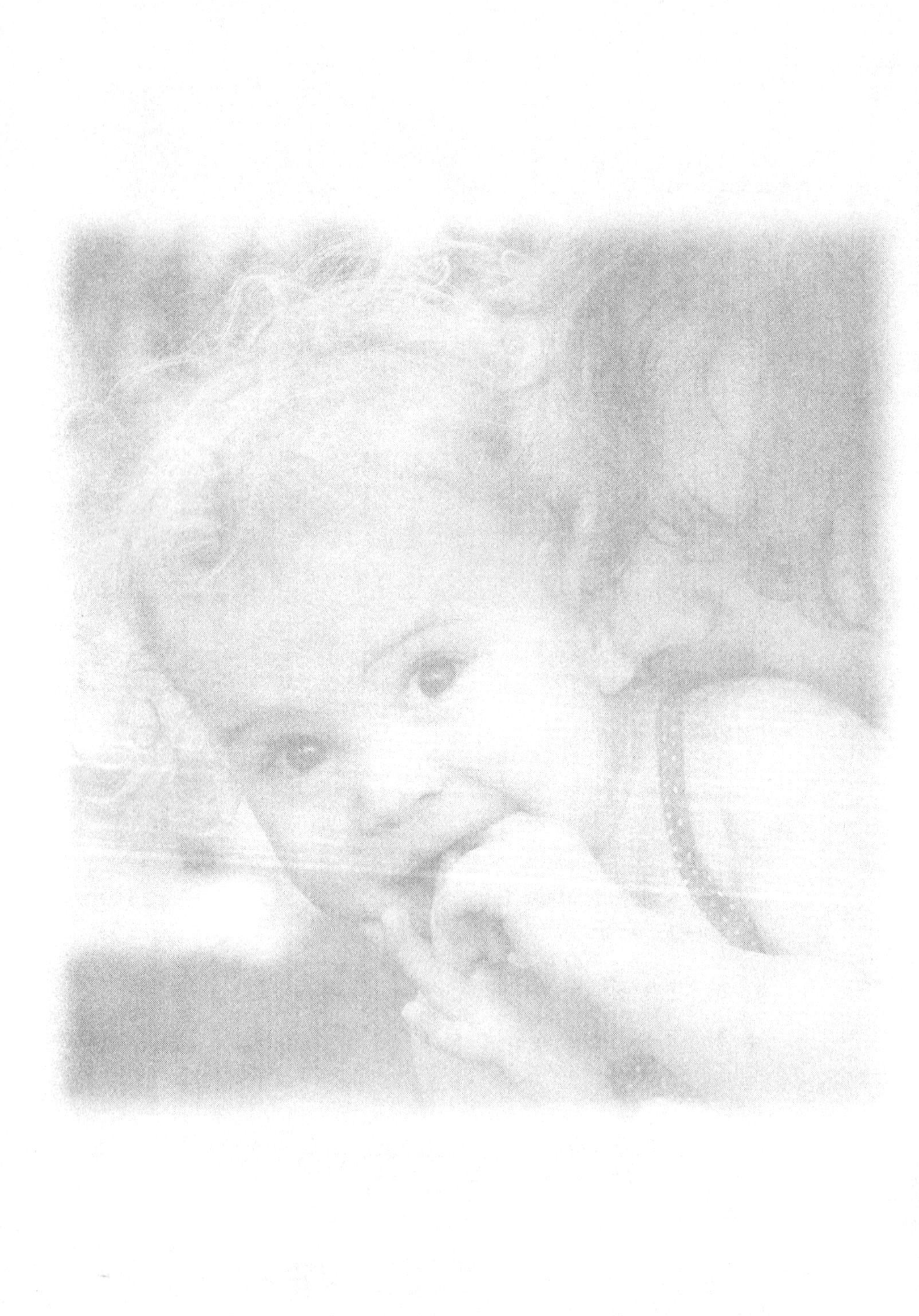

1— Do You Have Children?

*"Making the decision to have a child is momentous.
It is to decide forever to have your heart
go walking around outside your body." ~Elizabeth Stone*

"OK, class. This week's theme is *The Circus*! As we go into the gym, you can guide your toddlers to practice climbing up and down the stairs to reach the lions and monkeys or work on their balance by walking across the low balance beam. I will be over by the barrel helping the kids work on their spatial awareness as they crawl through."

This was a typical day at work.

I approached a new mom, previewing the class for the first time with her chubby 15-month old. Emily was just starting to work on her climbing skills so I went over to the small stairs to provide some assistance.

"Wow!" I said. "Emily is doing a great job climbing up those stairs. Just make sure she scoots down backwards, feet first, after she reaches the top."

"Really?" the mom replied. "She always goes down the stairs facing forward at home. Isn't that OK?"

"It's much safer for her to go down the stairs backwards," I said. "Sometimes they just need a little encouragement to learn how to do it safely. That's one of the best things about playing here. If they stumble, the padded floor and equipment will cushion the fall."

"Oh! That makes sense!" said the mom. "I guess you learn a lot about kids working in a place like this. Do you have kids?"

I paused, considering how to respond to her inquiry.

In 2007, my husband Roger and I had left the security of the workaday world and purchased a business. Our daughter, Charlotte, had gone to a summer camp for toddlers at a children's enrichment center near our home called *Romp n' Roll* and loved it. The business was local to our town but had begun franchising and one day, on a whim, Roger and I inquired with the corporate office as to what it would take to purchase our own location. The business capitalized on all our strengths and interests, and the timing was right for us financially. Six months after our initial letter of interest, we jumped off the proverbial ledge and purchased the location near our house from the original owners. We now ran a business that taught gym, art, and music classes to preschool-aged kids during the week and hosted birthday parties on the weekend. We weren't making a whole lot of money, but we loved our jobs.

Every day, I taught 45-minute gym and music classes for kids from the ages of 3 months to 6 years. Our program, which revolved around new themes each week, taught parents how to encourage their children's motor and language development through play. During the classes, the parents were able to talk to one another, sharing the joys and challenges of raising their children and offering support. As an instructor, I facilitated a lot of that interaction.

I thought of all the events of the last three years as I considered this mother's question. This was a business focused entirely around children. I was here because of my innate love for kids. More importantly, I owned this business because of our daughter's early experiences. This logical and perfectly innocuous question gave our conversation a whole new direction. This was a very common and natural question, but over the last few months, I had been struggling with how to answer it.

Today I said, "Not anymore. Not right now." The mom looked at me quizzically. She almost did a double take as she tried to comprehend what I said while keeping an eye on her toddling daughter. I explained, using the words I had practiced in my head over the last few months: "I had a daughter. She died of a brain tumor back in January."

Those were the words that kept me grounded in the present. This was the statement with which I greeted each new day. This is my reality.

Cancer attacked our world in January, 2009. Although it was my daughter who claimed the diagnosis, the disease devastated our entire family. We learned a lot by dealing with the cancer that mercilessly attacked us: how the hospital system works, the importance of patient advocacy, the kindness of strangers, and the depth of our personal strength. Before this experience, we hadn't really lived *cancer*. No one in either Roger's or my immediate

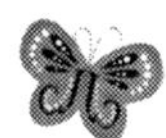

families had died from cancer, and we hadn't had many close friends who had fought the cancer battle. We certainly had never known any children who had struggled with something like this.

We faced the battle of a lifetime, one that blindsided us with an unimaginable force. We were ready to do anything for our daughter. During that year, we learned more than I ever could have expected about what it means to be a parent and what it means to lose your only child.

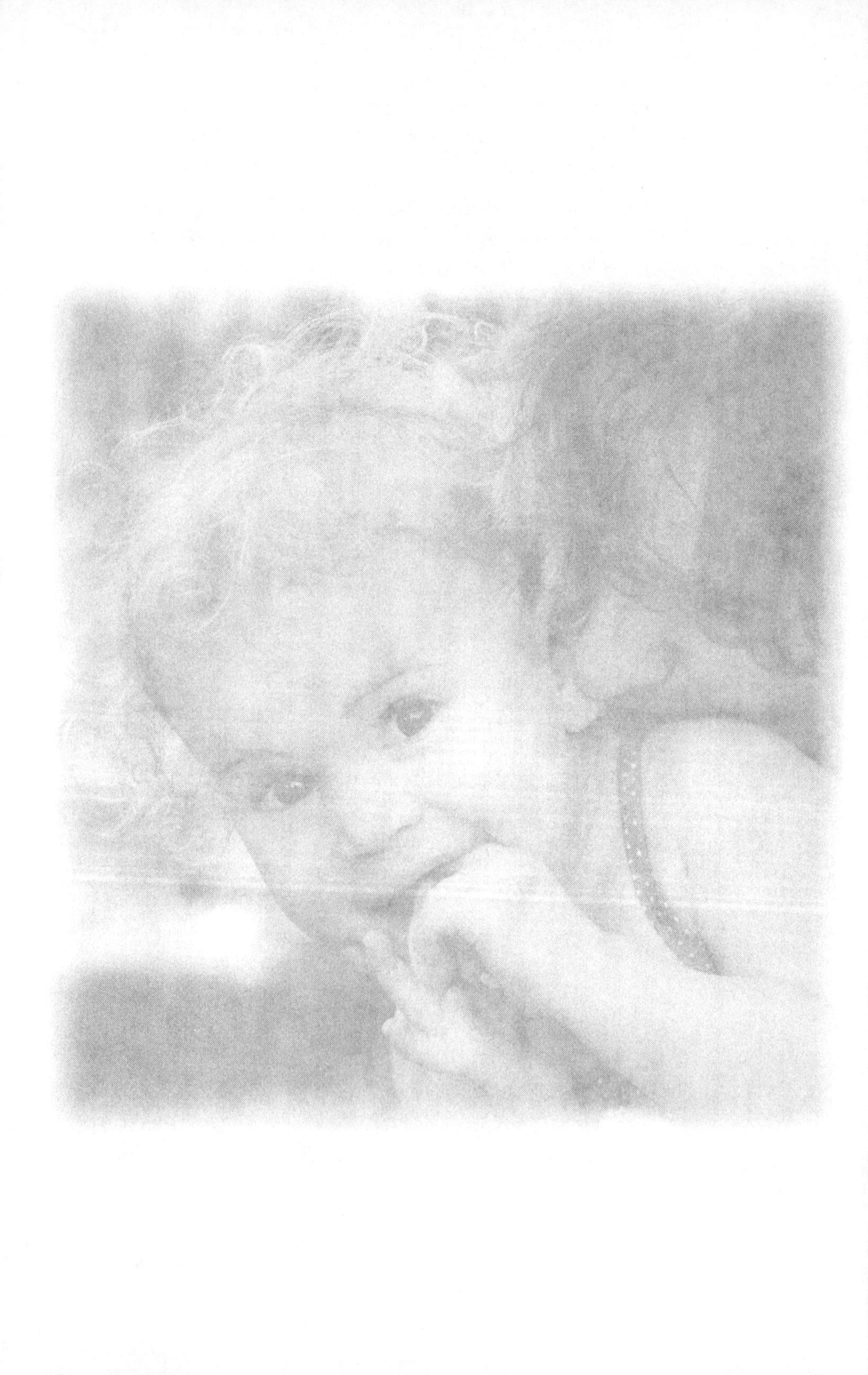

2— The Day Our Lives Changed Forever

My husband Roger is a runner. On his birthday in January 2001, after years of being out of the running habit, he set a goal to run his first marathon. He ran a mile that day and thought he was going to collapse. Despite his rocky start, he registered for the Marine Corps Marathon set for October of that year and began a training regimen. As the year continued, he added a few more miles to his training schedule each week. I also learned, as the year progressed, what it meant to be married to an athlete.

Weekends were now devoted to training for marathons. Roger registered for 10Ks, half-marathons, and 10-milers in our area as preparation for the big day. The races impacted our time together, and his new hobby also made a significant dent in our bank account. It wasn't just the race fees, either. He needed new shoes every 200 miles. Racing gear such as shirts, running shorts, body glide, energy bars, and sweat-wicking socks were all part of the running package. I started to count the days until we could put this marathon endeavor behind us.

No one would ever describe me as "athletic." I had no problem taking on the role of head cheerleader and pack mule, carting our gear from start line to finish line at each race, meeting up with Roger at designated points to help replenish fluids and sustenance during the long training runs, and cheering him on at every point along the journey. I found my place in our new "family hobby," but it wasn't exactly my cup of tea. When we talked with friends about Roger's new endeavor, they would frequently turn to me and say, "So, do you run too?" I always responded with a succinct but confident reply: "No. Running is not my thing. I'm just the cheerleader."

The day of the event finally arrived, and Roger told me, "My goal is to finish this run and if it's the only marathon I ever do, I will be happy." Five minutes after crossing the finish line, he was already planning his next marathon effort.

I resigned myself to my new role as the wife of a runner.

Although I was reluctant to embrace Roger's rekindled passion, I was incredibly proud of him. Running 26 miles was certainly a feat outside of my abilities. I found myself close to tears every time he crossed a new finish line and accomplished another goal. During each race, I found those strategic spots along the course where I could be there to cheer on Roger (and the other athletes), provide Ibuprofen and BioFreeze, and encourage him to keep going. This was my job and if you ask my husband, it's almost as important as running the course.

After that first marathon, Roger set a goal to run at least one marathon a year. On November 15, 2008, Roger ran his sixth marathon in our adopted hometown of Richmond, VA. On January 10, 2009, he ran his seventh marathon at Disney World. Ten days later, our eighth marathon started.

January 2010 had already been a busy month. Falling on the heels of a whirlwind holiday season, Roger and our three-year-old daughter, Charlotte, took a long weekend to Florida for the Disney Marathon. I was disappointed that responsibilities at Romp n' Roll kept me from traveling with them. One of the realities of business ownership meant that true family vacations were few and far between. While we had originally planned to make the Disney Marathon trip together, situations at work interfered and I stayed home to mind the store.

I had no worries about Charlotte traveling with her dad. At the age of three, she was already a seasoned traveler. Her first airplane trip came when she was only six months old. Charlotte slept a lot, nursed through the takeoffs and landings, and provided an almost-perfect traveling experience for us as first-time parents. Since we had family scattered all across the country, we ended up traveling via airplane almost every six months. I can't recall a single trip that was challenging (at least because of Charlotte). She was always easily entertained with books, movies, or a strategically revealed snack. We often heard comments from other passengers during our flights such as, "Oh, she's such a good baby," or "I didn't hear a peep out of her the entire flight. Was she asleep?" In short, I felt grateful that we had a child who traveled well.

While I was sad that I wasn't able to make the trip myself, I knew they would have a great time. Roger embraced fatherhood from the very beginning. He has always had an innate ability to engage children in a calming way. He could do this with other people's children, but he had a particular way of charming Charlotte. He rarely (if ever) raised his voice to her. When he needed her to do something important, he explained it in a way she could understand and Charlotte responded accordingly. His demeanor with our daughter, as it was with all kids, had an almost Zen quality to it. I knew that even if there were any challenges during their trip, Charlotte was in good hands with her daddy.

In addition to the marathon event, Charlotte was able to visit her Florida grandparents. We had been talking to Charlotte since Christmas about going to see Granny and Gramps. She was excited to see the beach again, even if it was January. Her grandparents spent the weeks leading up to the visit planning all kinds of outings to her favorite places, such as the library and the neighborhood parks.

I expected a phone call when they arrived in Florida, but I didn't expect the news that Roger shared when the phone rang.

"I think Charlotte might be getting sick," he said.

"Uh oh," I responded. "What's going on?"

"Well, she kept holding her ears and screaming every time the plane took off and landed. She's never done that before. She kind of has a fever too. It's low-grade, but we're keeping an eye on her. She actually threw up after we got off the plane," he said.

"Wow. That's weird," I responded. "Anything else?"

"Well, she definitely seems more tired than usual," Roger said. "She slept in the car as we drove from Orlando to your parents' house."

"Oh, I hope she's not getting that stomach bug that everyone at school seems to have," I said. "Just keep me updated, OK?"

I was a little bit worried, but work kept me distracted until their return from Florida. I pushed those symptoms to the back of my mind, convinced that it was nothing more than a small intestinal bug or a mild case of the flu.

After they got back from Florida, her symptoms persisted. We called the pediatrician the day after Roger and Charlotte returned and they saw her for a cursory sick visit. The stomach bug still seemed to be the obvious culprit. The nurse felt that she should be fine in a few days and told us to call if she wasn't better soon.

Charlotte had always been a relatively healthy kid. She got the usual minor sinus infections that made the rounds through preschool and daycare, but her bouts of sickness usually only lasted a few days. Rest, fluids, and sometimes a round of antibiotics were usually all we needed to make her feel better again.

This illness was different.

After returning from Florida, Charlotte started complaining that her head hurt. "Mommy, I need some medicine," she said to me.

"Medicine?" I asked. "Why do you need medicine?"

"My head hurts."

The first few times she said this, I gave her some Ibuprofen and tried to increase her fluid intake. I considered everything she had been through in the last few days. I figured she was probably just nursing a headache due to dehydration. Between the vomiting, the travel on multiple airplanes, and the dry January weather, fluids seemed to be an easy and immediate solution.

After a day or so of this behavior, though, she kept complaining of her head hurting and she continued to ask for medicine.

"Charlotte, *where* does your head hurt?" I finally asked.

"In the back," she said. I felt my body go numb for a moment. A tingle shot up my spine, but I stayed calm.

"In the back? Hmm. Could you show me where it hurts?" She pointed to the very back of her head, almost at the nape of her neck. I asked her the same question throughout the day and always got the same response. I began to get more concerned. Kids don't usually get headaches in the back of their head. Adults don't either, for that matter.

Then there were other symptoms. Charlotte was a wonderful child, but developing a good sleep routine was not a skill that she had mastered early in life. I spent many late nights rocking my infant daughter because she refused to align her body clock with a reasonable schedule of sleeping and waking. While most kids learn how to make it through the night without waking

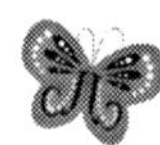

or crying sometime in the first year, Charlotte continued to wake almost every night until she was almost two years old. She was also not very good at napping during the day. When she was much younger, she would take a nap that lasted an hour or two. By the time she turned two, she dropped her mid-day nap altogether. I could always tell when she was getting sick because she would *finally* nap during the day. As she continued to complain about her headaches, she was snuggling up to us during the day, saying that she was sleepy and wanted to take a nap.

"Mommy, I'm tired," she said weakly.

"OK, sweetie," I responded. "Do you want to take a nap?"

"No. I just want to sit here with you. Is that OK?"

"Sure, honey. I need to work on this report, but you can lie here next to me on the couch if you want."

"OK, Mommy. I just want my headache to go away."

"I know, honey. Why don't you just rest your head in my lap?"

A few minutes later, she was asleep. I hadn't sent her to preschool since she returned from the Florida trip, wanting her to recover before sending her back. It had been over a week since her symptoms had started and she seemed to be getting worse, not better. This was far from normal, even for a child who might be fighting a stomach bug or the flu.

On Monday, I called the doctor's office again. I told the nurse about her symptoms and she seemed a little more concerned this time. It was about 3:00 p.m. so she said, "If she's not better by tomorrow, you should definitely call to have her come in."

That evening, I decided to call my mom. I always found her to be a reasonable anchor when I had questions about parenting or health related issues. Maybe she could help me keep all of this in perspective. "It just was so unusual," my mom said. "She would be fine during the day, but every morning and every night, she would throw up. We kept thinking it was just effects of the flight, but even a few days after she got here, she kept having troubles."

"I know, Mom. She's been complaining about her head hurting. It's really weird because she says her head hurts in the back. Don't you think that's weird? I mean, headaches don't usually hurt in the back of the head like that."

My mom was really quiet for a few minutes. "Mom, what is it?"

Finally, she took a deep breath and said, "You know, William was having headaches like that before he got sick."

William is my godmother's nephew. He was diagnosed with Leukemia in 2005 and had been receiving treatments at St. Jude Children's Hospital in Tennessee. After a long treatment regimen, William is now healthy and doing very well, but I remembered how stressful that had been for my godmother's family. I quickly pushed my mother's thoughts out of my head. "Mom, she's probably fine. I don't think that could be it. Really? She's a healthy kid. I think she's just having trouble recovering from the trip to Florida. Roger's going to take her to the doctor in the morning."

"You're probably right," my mom said. "Let me know when you get some news."

Roger took her in to the doctor about 8:30 a.m. on Tuesday. He had the morning off anyway and wasn't scheduled to be at Romp n' Roll until the afternoon shift of classes. I, meanwhile, went off to work. I had a full morning of teaching classes at Romp n' Roll. I mentioned to our manager that I was expecting a call from Roger since he was taking Charlotte to the doctor. Every time a class ended, I used my mini-break to check my phone, looking for a text message or voicemail that would give me some news. By the time the third class finished around noon, I was full of nervous energy.

It was already an exciting day, an historic day. It was January 20, 2009. We had a new President taking the oath of office. While we didn't have a television at the store, I planned to watch the Inaugural Address on my computer as soon as my last morning class was over. I was trying desperately to take in everything surrounding this historic moment, but my thoughts kept wandering to Charlotte. Why hadn't Roger called? Their appointment was almost four hours ago. Why wasn't there any news?

My cell phone finally rang just as President Obama was finishing his Inaugural remarks. "Finally," I thought. "Now I can find out what's going on and we can go get some lunch together." Roger relayed the news in his usual matter-of-fact way. When it comes to emergencies, he is always the least likely to be rattled. Even still, I could hear the tension that he tried to disguise in his voice: "Hi, Rachel. We have been at the emergency room. She had a CT scan. They've found something. We're going directly to another hospital and I'm coming to get you right now. Shall I get you some lunch?"

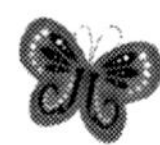

My first thought was that conversation I'd had barely 24 hours before with my mother. Is this serious? Is she sick? Is this more than just the stomach flu? All I remember saying was, "OK." I couldn't think of what to do next.

I packed up my belongings, got our manager to start working on afternoon coverage in case Roger wasn't available to teach his classes, and ran to the car when he pulled up outside the store. I could see the concern in his eyes, but he still seemed very calm. I looked at Charlotte in her car seat. She was awake but looked tired. "Hi, Mommy," was all she said.

Roger and I were both worried. We weren't quite sure how to process the information yet. The last thing on my mind was food, but since we didn't know what the rest of the afternoon would hold, we stopped at the Chick-Fil-A drive-through to get something to bring to the hospital. While we waited in the queue, Roger provided more details about the last few hours with the doctors. "The pediatrician was concerned when he examined Charlotte's eyes," he said. "There was something about fluid or pressure. Dr. Weber sent us to St. Mary's for a CT scan. That's when they found a mass in her head. The doctor in the ER said it wasn't very big. We have to go to another hospital for an MRI and a meeting with a doctor there."

As he told me all of this information, I kept turning in my seat to look at Charlotte. Did she understand anything that her dad and I were discussing? She didn't seem upset and that calmed me. All I could think about was that conversation I had with my mother the day before. I didn't call her yet. I needed more information. I needed to know what was wrong. Charlotte looked back at me and smiled weakly.

We arrived at VCU Medical Center (also known as MCV) fairly quickly. MCV is Richmond's largest hospital and home to Virginia Commonwealth University's medical school. Roger had been given some vague and rudimentary directions by the people in the emergency room. Once we were able to park, we navigated our way through three different buildings, using two different elevators, to the sixth floor of the Ambulatory Care Clinic. Until we got there, I didn't realize that we had been directed to the Office of Neurosurgery. It seemed like any other doctor's office. The fact that we hadn't been rushed immediately to another emergency room was somehow calming to me. I rationalized that if there was something *truly* wrong with Charlotte, they wouldn't just send us to another specialist. Whatever was wrong, this was where we would find a solution. Perhaps we would get a diagnosis and they would see us for a follow up appointment in a week. This thought process was the only thing that reassured me at that point.

A receptionist greeted us and took the pile of paperwork that we had been given earlier that day. We checked in, handed over the requisite insurance cards and other information and waited. We had a file folder containing her scan from the ER on a CD and that was it. The fear of the unknown began to creep in slowly. What we wanted was information and all we could do was wait.

We tried to eat, but our appetite was pretty much shot. I knew that I was hungry. I hadn't had anything to eat since breakfast and neither had Roger. The French fries just sat in the bag, getting colder and less appetizing by the minute. I enticed Charlotte to eat a few chicken nuggets, usually one of her favorite foods, but she didn't seem interested in food either.

Charlotte was newly potty trained so we would check with her about every hour.

"Do you need to go potty?"

"Yes, Mommy," she'd say. We would go off to the closest bathroom in an effort to avoid an accident. As in so many situations, she was pleasant and easily entertained. She just sat as we read her books or played games. "When are we going to see the doctor, Daddy?" she asked.

"Soon," he said absentmindedly.

"Mommy, will you read this book to me?"

"Sure, honey. Why don't you tell me about the kids in this picture?" I was grateful that keeping Charlotte occupied was rarely a challenge because I was definitely distracted.

Finally, we were escorted back to one of the patient rooms where we met Joanne, a nurse practitioner with a pleasant demeanor and a kind spirit. She said a few words to Charlotte, "Hey sweetie. What's your name?"

"Charlotte Jennie Reynolds," she said, without missing a beat.

"Oh, aren't you a cutie. Are you feeling OK?" Joanne asked.

"My head hurts," Charlotte said.

"Really?" said Joanne. "Where does it hurt, honey?" While she asked these questions to Charlotte, Joanne kept looking to Roger and me for confirmation.

 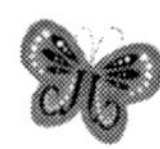

"In the back," she said and pointed to that same spot that she had indicated over the past three days.

"Well," Joanne said, "I'm going to take this scan over to the office and Dr. Tye should be here in just a few minutes to meet with you." She gave all three of us a reassuring smile and left us to sit and wait.

About 15 minutes passed before we met Dr. Gary Tye. He wore a neat pin-striped Oxford shirt with a coordinating tie. He looked like he had stepped into our exam room from the cover of *GQ* magazine instead of the halls of the hospital. What immediately impressed me about Dr. Tye was the way he made eye contact with all three of us upon entering the room. I could tell that he had a busy practice and frequently rushed from one patient or procedure to another. At the same time, I immediately had a sense that, at that very moment, we were his most important patients.

He brought the scan into the room and installed the CD on a computer there. He started to bring up the image on the monitor while making some small talk, introducing himself, and asking questions about Charlotte's recent behavior. Roger and I recounted the same story we had been telling for the past week: the airplane trips, the vomiting, the sleepiness, the reports of headaches. Dr. Tye was asking more questions: Was she having trouble walking? Had there been any seizures? How long had we seen these symptoms? I stopped hearing the questions once I saw *IT*.

The mass.

Already, my parental instincts had told me that something was wrong. The brain scan simply confirmed my worst fear. This was not the scan of a healthy brain. There was this very large mass in the middle of her head. It seemed to take up almost her entire skull.

"That's not tiny," I said softly.

Dr. Tye looked straight into my eyes and said, "No, it's not."

While the details of that moment will probably always be fuzzy, the reality of our next step was clear: Charlotte was not going home. We were waiting to be admitted to the Pediatric Intensive Care Unit (PICU).

So we waited. In the meantime, Roger and I started calling family and friends. We knew that we were now in a serious situation, but we didn't have a lot of information ourselves. I braced myself for the onslaught of unanswerable questions. One of the first people I called was my friend, Melissa. She was a music therapist working at the hospital and I thought she might still be at work.

"Hello?" she answered.

"Melissa? It's Rachel."

"Oh, hey! What's going on?"

"Are you at work?"

"No. We are in D.C.! We went to the Inauguration. It was so exciting! We just stepped out of the Metro."

"Oh! I'm so sorry! I'll try to catch up with you later," I said.

"Well, wait! What's going on?"

"It's Charlotte," I said. "They're admitting her to the PICU right now. They found something in her head. It might be a tumor."

I said those words. I said them out loud for the very first time. Now there was no denying the reality of the situation.

"Wait! What? Really? Oh, Rachel! I'll be there first thing tomorrow morning. I'll come find you, OK? Is there anything you need right now?"

"No," I said, holding back the first of many tears. "I'll see you tomorrow. Thanks."

Roger and I repeated a variation of this conversation at least 50 times that evening. We called our family, most of whom were far away in other states and time zones. We called close friends. We called our pastor. We called our employees to arrange coverage for the next few days. Finally, I called my mother, taking a deep breath as I needed to confirm her worst fear.

"Mom, it's me. Charlotte's OK right now, but I need to let you know they found something in her head. It might be a tumor. They're admitting us to the ICU tonight."

"Oh my. Oh dear. Oh no." My mother's anxiety came through the phone and I could picture her face, fraught with worry. "What are they going to do?"

"We don't know yet," I tried to say in as calm a voice as I could muster. "They're going to do more tests tomorrow, but it looks like she might need to have surgery. I'm staying with her tonight. I'll call you as soon as we have more news. I promise."

We called Auntie 'Retta, Charlotte's godmother, who came almost as soon as she heard, arriving shortly after we were finally admitted to the PICU. A mom of two boys herself, Loretta brought things that she knew would distract Charlotte: a few books, a stuffed rabbit, and some coloring pages. The evening consisted of settling Charlotte into a strange bed, hooking her up to monitors and taking vitals. Charlotte was happy to have books to read, but didn't seem too interested in the crayons. Since she had never had much of a "lovey" or favorite toy, we just kept her interested in items that we found closest to us. She was still really tired so she kept falling asleep as Loretta and I read a few stories to pass the time.

I didn't sleep much that first night in the hospital. Roger had gone home to take care of things and promised to be back in the morning in time for her MRI.

The next day, Charlotte's health really started to go downhill.

"Mom, my head still hurts," she said in the morning.

"I'm sorry, Charlotte. That's why we're here. The doctors are trying to figure out how to make your head feel better."

"What are they going to do?"

"Well, you're going to have a test this morning. They're going to take a picture of your head and see if they can figure out what is wrong."

"Oh," she said and went back to watching *Curious George* on television.

Normally, I would have expected more questions from Charlotte. She was an inquisitive kid who was always asking about current events and trying to figure out what was going on. As the day progressed, however, she simply became more and more lethargic. She kept asking to go to sleep or watch television. I decided to just let her rest.

The worst-case scenarios kept running through my head. Since we were admitted to the PICU, Charlotte had to be hooked up to machines that monitored her heart rate, pulse, and oxygen levels. On the one hand, this was reassuring because I knew that if anything started to go horribly wrong, the doctors and nurses would know in a moment that she was in trouble. At the same time, I kept thinking about the upcoming MRI and the surgery that Dr. Tye had promised was almost certainly a part of Charlotte's near future. At this point, all I wanted was answers. I couldn't stand living in the ambiguity of the unknown.

By the time the medical personnel came to transport Charlotte down to the MRI room, all we could do was follow. Roger tried to prepare Charlotte for what was about to happen.

"Charlotte, we're riding down in the elevator because they are going to take another picture of your brain."

"Really?" she said, wide-eyed with amazement.

The previous day's CT scan at the emergency room was a rough experience. Charlotte was alright as Roger laid her down on the scanning bed, but as soon as her head was on the scanner, she started crying and screaming.

"It hurts! It hurts!" Charlotte said.

"What hurts?" Roger responded.

"My head. I want to get up!"

"You can't get up," Roger tried to reassure her. "I'll be right here. I'm not going anywhere. You just need to lie still for a minute."

"No! It hurts!"

At this point, the radiology tech came over and tried to help. "She says it's hurting her head," Roger said to him.

"Well, it shouldn't hurt her head at all. We need her to lie still, OK? Do you want to sit with her and help her?"

Roger was draped in a lead mat to block the radiation and held Charlotte's chin up while they completed the CT scan the day before. Fortunately, it was a quick process and once it was over, she was calm again. This time, however, we wouldn't be able to sit with her during the MRI. Roger just kept repeating the process to her in a calm voice, "They're going to give you some gas to help you take a nap. Then they are going to take a picture of your brain while you sleep." Charlotte just kept nodding weakly.

It was difficult to reassure her when we were, ourselves, terrified of the great big unknown we were facing. The mystery compounded itself with big scary signs in the radiology waiting area warning everyone to make sure all metal was emptied from your pockets and all jewelry was removed before entering the room. One of us, probably me, shakily completed an exhaustive pre-procedure checklist inquiring about previous medical procedures, implants, medical conditions, and all kinds of medical information.

Roger actually took Charlotte into the MRI room and the techs gave him the mask that would deliver the anesthesia. When Charlotte was two, she had been sick with a mild case of walking pneumonia. To help with her breathing, she had been prescribed a treatment using masks with cute little animals on them. Despite the novelty, she had hated it and fought the process every time we tried to get her to use the Nebulizer.

This time was no exception and it was very difficult for Roger to get the mask over her face.

"Charlotte, you need to put the mask on so you can go to sleep."

"No!" she yelled as she shook her head back and forth. "No! No! No! I don't want to."

"I know you don't, Charlotte, but this is what the doctors need to do to take a picture of your head."

Fortunately, her crying actually helped the process along because the gas was inhaled more quickly. Within a few short minutes, the anesthesiologist had done her job and the radiologist could begin the scan of her brain.

When we finally closed the door and they started the MRI, Roger and I both collapsed. We cried on each other's shoulders, seeming to realize just in this moment that *this was a matter of life and death*. This was the first time I remember actually crying since we had started the sequence of events that led us from the pediatrician's office to the emergency room to the neurosurgeon's office and finally to the PICU. This was the first time that we really stopped and considered her mortality in all of this. She could die. Whatever this thing was in her head could *kill* her. Although I was anxious for the answers the MRI would provide, I was also terrified of what they would find and what those findings would mean for our lives.

The MRI results revealed a very large tumor (about the size of a large orange) in the middle of her brain. It was a rare and aggressive form of cancer known as PNET: Primitive Neuroectodermal Tumor. It was filling the cavity above the thalamus that would normally contain spinal fluid. The tumor was putting pressure on the fluid in the ventricles, which was causing the swelling and pain. Given its size and placement, the doctors were amazed that she was as functional and asymptomatic as she was on her admission to the hospital. Many times, these types of tumors can go undetected until they cause seizures or a brain hemorrhage. According to the neurosurgeon, the tumor touched some very important parts of her brain.

Surgery was scheduled for 8:30 the next morning. We made more phone calls, contacting almost everyone in our address book as we had the day before. Charlotte remained lethargic, sleeping much of the time. She didn't eat much and she never even asked to get out of bed. At one point, Roger tried to explain the surgery to her.

"Charlotte, they found a tumor in your head. That is what is making your head hurt. Tomorrow, you're going to take a long nap and Dr. Tye is going to try to take it out. We hope that will make your headache go away."

"OK, Daddy," was all Charlotte said. She looked at him with her big brown eyes. Even at three years of age, she seemed to understand. If she didn't understand, she at least trusted that we would keep her safe.

My focus was gone. When I wasn't sitting with Charlotte in her hospital room, I was making phone calls, pacing the floor, and trying to calm my anxious brain. In less than two days, our world had been turned upside-down. Nothing was right. Nothing felt safe.

As I sat in the family room on the pediatric unit, waiting for family coming in from out-of-town, I looked around, fixing my gaze on a beach scene hanging on the wall. I thought of the warmth of the sun, the calming lull of the waves. The image reminded me of South Florida, where Roger and I first met. That happy place was a world away right now.

3— Hospital Time

If someone had walked up to me on the day that Roger and I met and said, "This is the man you are going to marry," I would have questioned that person's sanity. I was a straight-laced freshman at the University of Miami. Roger was a hip graduate student majoring in Jazz Studies with long hair, a dangly earring, and wild clothes. We couldn't have been more different from one another. Plus, I had a boyfriend at the time, the kind of boyfriend I thought I was going to marry. We had been together for almost three years and had already discussed settling down after I finished college. I was on my way to the prototypical marriage -- a house with a white picket fence, 2.5 kids, and a dog.

Thanks to our mutual involvement in the music fraternities on campus, Roger and I ended up floating in the same social circles. My best friend, Rebecca, was also one of Roger's good friends. They met the year before when her high school visited the University of Miami on a tour. By my second year of college, I had ended my relationship with my high school boyfriend and my friendship with Roger had grown closer. We soon found ourselves inseparable. We quickly became one of those couples who finish each other's sentences.

By my senior year in 1997, Roger had finished his Masters Degree and was working in a teacher's exchange program in South Korea. Although the initial idea of the two of us together had seemed illogical, time had a way of changing things. Now we couldn't stand the idea of living apart. He surprised me with a ring during a Christmas visit and I counted the days until he returned to the United States.

This was back before email was widespread and the bulk of our long-distance correspondence was in the form of hand-written letters. We wrote to one another, across the miles, planning our wedding, searching for jobs, and talking about our plans to start a family in our new home, wherever that might be.

I was born and raised in Florida, but Roger was raised in Illinois and Colorado. We were both ready to leave Florida for a while, so I sought out an internship, the final step in my Music Therapy degree, in locations where we could actually experience all four seasons.

Florida is unique for all kinds of reasons, but South Florida is an experience unto itself. The culture and the climate create a world unlike anything I've ever experienced. Events in South Florida rarely start on time and the phenomenon is known locally as *Cuban Time*. Maybe it's the humid, tropical air that makes time seem to pass in a different way. If you invite your guests to a party to at 8:00 p.m., it really won't get going until 10:00 or so. If a concert is set to start at 2:00 p.m., it isn't uncommon for it to commence around 2:15 or even 2:30. It is just understood. When this happens, you don't look at it as being late. Miami runs on *Cuban Time*. That's simply how it is. Those of us who relocate to the tropics, and live there long enough, just learn to adapt.

> Keep a notebook or journal handy so you can write notes about doctor's orders or medication changes. It's easy to forget these things.

In a similar manner, medical facilities run on *Hospital Time*. You learn quickly that appointments, procedures, rounds, medical orders, all of these things that are necessary for your child, just happen when they happen. The time when they *say* something will happen is only a guideline. Your MRI is scheduled for 8:00 a.m.? You'll probably go in for the procedure around 8:45. You are supposed to be admitted to the hospital on Friday? You'll get there first thing in the morning for tests and admitting procedures, but you won't be admitted to your room until about 5:00 p.m.-- if you're lucky. Dinner is served between 5:30 and 6 p.m.? Well, if the nurse forgot to remove your child's "no food" order that was in place earlier in the day due to her CT scan, the meal

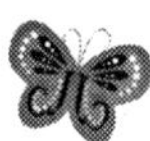

cart will skip your child's room and she won't get another meal until next morning's breakfast (unless you go out and forage for some food on your own).

On January 20, 2009, we started a crash course in the hospital system from a parent's point of view. We were thrust into a world with new terminology, unfamiliar people, and a unique set of rules. There were rules about when and where we could use our cell phones, rules for visiting hours, rules for who could administer medications. There were forms to fill out every time I turned around; I had to show our insurance card at every twist and turn in the process. I was faced with terms like "malignant tumor," "hematocrit levels" and "infusion of cisplatin." Although our first instinct was to trust the medical professionals, we also felt this incredible need to understand everything going on around us.

Visits to and from the hospital became as routine as trips to the grocery store. Our leisure time was now relegated to sharing a movie with our daughter from her hospital bed. Our personal conversations were constantly interrupted by beeping machines, medical rounds by the doctors, or the administration of new medications as they were added to Charlotte's IV.

Keep in mind that we had nothing but the utmost respect for Charlotte's doctors and the nurses who worked with us in the pediatric oncology clinic, as well as the inpatient areas. We received care from two fabulous hospitals over the course of a year. We rarely found complaint with the quality of staff.

Efficient communication and effective service delivery, however, were often quite another matter.

We would sometimes show up to the clinic only to find out they "didn't have an appointment made" for her. **Lesson learned:** *we would call the clinic as soon as we left our house so that our nurse could order her medications.* By the time we reached the hospital (about 30 minutes later), our medications were either waiting for us or at least ordered and in process.

Other days, the clinic was just *full* of patients and what should have been a 30-minute visit turned into a 60-minute wait in the lobby and a 90- minute additional wait in the clinic. **Lesson learned:** *we came prepared with plenty of books, movies, or other activities for both Charlotte and ourselves.* Through all of these procedures, Charlotte was probably the most tolerant of all of us. She had always been a kid who could *go with the flow.* As long as she had a few books to look at or a movie to watch, Charlotte was happy. She was what I liked to call a *serial monogamist.* She would like a show or a book and read it over… and over… and over again. Then she would find a new favorite and the cycle would start anew.

I remember reading the book *Brown Bear, Brown Bear* so often on a road trip to Colorado, that I could recite the story from memory. Charlotte was barely a year old at the time, but she would say, "Again, Mommy." When we visited the clinic, we often brought our portable DVD player. The clinic and the hospital had lots of videos available for the kids, but we never knew if her "latest favorite" would be in use by another patient or broken or lost. We traveled with a plentiful supply of *Curious George, Dora the Explorer,* and just about any Disney movie ever made. If she had a video to watch, Charlotte was usually pretty happy.

Always expect that you will have to wait. Bring books, movies, or video games to keep you or your child entertained.

Probably one of the most frustrating situations would be when Charlotte would have NPO orders *(Nil Per Oral),* meaning she couldn't eat or drink anything. This would typically happen before procedures like MRIs, surgery, or radiation where she needed to be sedated. The goal was to always schedule NPO appointments first thing in the morning to minimize the amount of time she would have to go without food.

Unfortunately, *Hospital Time* is always unpredictable. On at least two occasions, we were scheduled for an MRI only to have delay upon delay. Next thing we knew, it was 1 p.m. and Charlotte had yet to eat or drink anything. When we started proton therapy, the schedule was already full of pediatric patients and her earliest appointment was 3 p.m.

The proton center ran on its own timetable. It has sensitive equipment that requires specialized software and a proton accelerator that mimics a nuclear reactor. The entire building would sometimes have to shut down when the equipment hit a glitch of one kind or another. It was usual, if not expected, to have delays at the proton center of an hour or more.

When Charlotte started proton radiation treatments, Roger was the first parent "on duty" to take her to the clinic. Before the course of radiation started, we had already spent a week hopping between diagnostic appointments, scans, and clinic visits, getting everything ready for these new procedures. Things seemed to actually be going relatively well until the first day of the actual proton radiation. The moment they got to the proton center, things started going wrong. Upon signing in, it was announced to the small group of patients that things were backed up and a delay of at least an hour could be expected.

That was about as far as the customer service aspect of things went that day. Roger's frustrations mounted, revolving around Charlotte's NPO status, as they waited and waited and waited, all with little or no word about how things were going. Roger was getting more and more irate at the staff for not informing him of how things were progressing. The final straw was when one of the health professionals came out of the treatment area with a box of chocolates and proceeded to go around the waiting area, asking everyone if they would like a piece, including kids like Charlotte who were not allowed to eat or drink.

Roger nearly flipped his lid and finally demanded loudly to anyone in a lab coat that either they were going to take Charlotte in or he was going to have to give her something to eat. By this time, it was creeping into late afternoon and neither of them had had anything to eat for going on 20 hours.

Someone took pity on Roger as a squeaky wheel and at least got Charlotte into a "prep" room. When they finally called Charlotte in for radiation at almost 5:00 p.m. for a 2:00/2:30/3:30 p.m. appointment (depending on which schedule you checked) Roger wanted nothing to do with the staff and all attempts the radiology and nursing crew made to comfort Charlotte just fell flat. "I didn't want to talk to anyone," he told me. "I just wanted to tell them to give her the 'goofy juice' and get out of there as quickly as possible before I blew a gasket!"

To top off an already terrible day, no one informed Roger when Charlotte emerged from radiation to the recovery room and by the time he heard any news, she was already waking up (alone). To this day it's one of his worst memories of the whole experience. And it all revolved around *Hospital Time*.

Of course, *Hospital Time* could very easily run the other way as well. Rarely (but enough that it threw us for a loop) a cancellation would occur and Charlotte would get pulled for a surgical procedure or MRI hours earlier than expected. You would think that this would be a good thing, but being awakened at 3:00 a.m. to be told that your daughter is going in for brain surgery at 6:00 a.m. instead of 8:00 a.m. is not necessarily welcome news. It sends your already anxious and sleep-deprived mind into overdrive.

How much time did we spend in the hospital? Charlotte was admitted to MCV on January 20 and was released (two brain surgeries later) on March 3rd. She spent over six weeks in the hospital during that first stretch. Four weeks later, we were admitted for a week's worth of inpatient chemotherapy. We checked out on a Friday only to be re-admitted four days later for a neutropenic fever. This resulted in another week-long hospital stay. We came home for about two more weeks and then checked in for round two of chemotherapy. This was another week in the hospital, thankfully out by Easter. We were admitted again less than a week later for another fever. During this round, we went in and out of the hospital twice due to fevers and infections. During round three, we calculated that our time in the hospital had substantially outnumbered our time at home. In three months, we had spent over 45 days admitted to the hospital. That didn't even count all the clinic and therapy visits that happened in-between hospital stays.

> **When you are going in and out of the hospital, keep a permanent list of the things you always need during your stay. It will help you remember handy items like lip balm and lotion.**

I have never been much of a frequent flier. I travel on occasion when necessary for business, but rarely stay overnight on these types of trips. There are those, however, whose jobs revolve around the constant routine of traveling for business (whether by plane, train, or automobile). When traveling, it is easy to spot the frequent fliers. They are the ones with the efficiently packed matching luggage. They breeze through security with an air of importance, mainly because they know the routine so well they can do it with their eyes closed. Frequent fliers know which airports have the best food courts. They know how to keep themselves occupied in case of delays. They always travel with a pair of backup clothes, just in case their luggage gets lost. In short, they know the system and they work it to their advantage.

We became "frequent fliers" in the hospital system. I began to wish the hospitals would give you little bar-coded key tags like you get at the grocery store. They could just save all of my information in their files and then, when they needed us to check in all over again, they could just scan the bar code.

 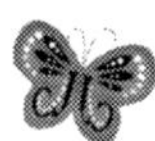

It would have saved on a lot of redundant paperwork and procedure. We became old pros at navigating the parking decks and negotiating security. We knew most of the security guards by name...or they at least recognized us. I remembered where the turtle statue was that Charlotte had to visit every time we passed through the Gateway building. I could find the quickest route to Chick-Fil-A from any point in the hospital. I knew which outdoor lunch carts offered the healthiest (and yummiest) meals, and the best times to avoid the crowds and the lines. The coffee cart guys remembered my order before I even asked for it, and didn't bat an eye when I was getting my 7:00 a.m. coffee in my pajamas.

Living in the hospital was not fun. Roger and I tried as much as possible to take turns so that we each got a decent night's sleep in our own bed at least *every other* night. A few times, Charlotte's grandparents even volunteered for an overnight stay so that Roger and I could have some time together outside of the hospital. Some of the rooms had pull-out beds that were reasonable (that's a kind term); however, many of the rooms had these reclining chairs that always reminded me of a Lucille Ball comedy sketch:

Step 1: Lie in the chair.

Step 2: Position your pillows and sheets: One pillow goes behind your head, another pillow goes behind your lower back. Cover yourself with at least one sheet. You may want to add a blanket if the hospital room is incredibly cold.

Step 3: Lean back in the chair to recline.

Step 4: *Don't move!* If you turn your head or shift your body in the slightest way, the chair will pop back up or your pillows will fall out from underneath you.

Step 5: Repeat steps 1-4 every 20-30 minutes. Inevitably your arm or leg will wake you with a cramp from lying in a strange position, or an IV monitor will start beeping, or a doctor or nurse will enter the room needing to check on medication levels or vitals.

It was ridiculous. Only those in a drug-induced sleep could get something resembling rest. Amazingly, Charlotte usually rested well during her hospital stays. She was one of those kids that could go back to sleep even when you nudged or poked her. Aside from the barrage of procedures (oh, and the fact that she was being injected with toxic chemicals), she usually weathered the stays in the hospital better than her parents did.

> Dress in layers. Temperature control in
> the hospital is practically nonexistent. It's
> usually too hot or too cold.

Eating in the hospital was another experience all unto itself. There is a reason why hospital food gets a bad rap. Charlotte's meals were pretty bland and generally overcooked. The fresh fruit and desserts were usually the best part. Options for the parents of patients were limited to McDonalds, the Bagel Place, Chick-Fil-A, the very limited cafeteria, and quite possibly the slowest Subway on the planet. None of the options were horrible in and of themselves, but day after day of these food choices got very old. We had some wonderful families deliver meals and snacks to us and we consumed a steady diet of frozen dinners, ready-to-eat soups, and the occasional delivered pizza or Chinese food. In short, it was a challenge to eat healthy. It didn't help that we usually craved yummy and highly caloric comfort food, and we could never seem to get enough caffeine.

As we navigated our new world, we got to know a host of new professionals who worked with us to make our life easier. Of course, there were the doctors and the nurses. We also worked with departments such as speech therapy, occupational therapy, and physical therapy as Charlotte recovered from the physical effects of brain surgery. Social workers, chaplains, and counselors attended to our mental health and provided a neutral shoulder to lean on when the stress proved overwhelming. I think the professionals that we looked forward to the most, though, were the members of the Child Life team.

The Child Life Department is every hospital's secret treasure. Their job is to help the patients, their siblings, and their parents weather the hospital experience by providing small perks and little comforts. This takes many forms. Their office is full of toys, games, videos, and art projects for children of all ages. They deliver these items to the pediatric hospital rooms during the day. Child Life also maintains the playrooms on the pediatric floor with age-appropriate toys and activities. Sometimes they host organized activities, usually facilitated by volunteers. During the holidays, Child Life would be responsible for helping volunteers deliver festive presents. They facilitated visits from therapy dogs, costumed cartoon characters, and local celebrities who try to brighten each patient's day.

Sometimes Child Life also helped to provide adaptive activities. After Charlotte's first surgery, one of the Child Life specialists came to our room with a lapboard, some shaving cream, and paint. When Charlotte's mobility was limited, this was a great activity and she had so much fun mixing the colored shaving cream and then wiping it all over her daddy's head!

Child Life also helped us as parents when we wondered how to explain medical procedures and other difficult concepts to our daughter. Knowing the ins and outs of the hospital experience, they answered our questions with regard to the next steps in a process. When do you think we are going to be discharged? What kind of follow-up can we expect from the doctor? If she comes in with a fever, are we going to be stuck here for a week? Do you know what time the cafeteria closes tonight? The people in Child Life either knew the answers or knew who to call.

When we finally were able to go home at the end of a hospital stay, they would help us pack all our belongings and provide wagons or carts so we could take our accumulated stuff across the many buildings and elevators to our car in the parking garage.

We became such regular fixtures at the hospital that the Child Life department knew us by name. They learned Charlotte's favorite movies and cartoon characters. When they would see Charlotte's name on an admission list, they would prepare her room ahead of time. During our fifth or sixth admission, we entered our appointed hospital room to find a stack of *Wonder Pets* DVDs already waiting for us with a pink and purple pillowcase on the bed, some new books waiting to be read, and a collection of little Care Bear figurines lined up on the shelf.

The Care Bears were a special link between Charlotte and her favorite Child Life specialist, Heather. Heather was one of the first people we met in the PICU, and she and Charlotte became instant buddies. One day, not long after her first surgery, Heather brought the Care Bears to visit Charlotte. The small three-inch plastic figurines were just the right size for Charlotte's little hands. They could sit on her hospital tray and keep her company. Sometimes she would say things like, "Grumpy Bear is blue." or "The pink bear is my favorite." She never really played with the bears or made up stories about them. She just liked to look at them and know that they were there. Heather brought them to her room during each hospital visit, always stressing that the Care Bears came to visit, not to stay. It was something for Charlotte to *borrow,* not to keep. Heather told me later, during our second or third stay in the hospital, "These kids get a lot of gifts while they are in the hospital. They get a lot of things that belong to them, but they don't get a lot of opportunities to share. Sometimes they need to remember the importance of sharing. That's why I let the kids 'borrow' some of my toys while they are here."

The Care Bear visit was also a constant ritual in a world that seemed to change from one hour to the next. Thanks to Child Life, Charlotte had a steady stream of entertainment at all times. She was pretty much contained to a bed except for occasional rides that she could take in a wagon, so DVDs of favorite TV shows and movies played frequently. Sometimes we were able to engage her in simple games like Candy Land or some craft activities. She loved to place stickers all over a paper and then make scenes out of the sticker designs. Even though she didn't always have the fine motor skills to move her arms and hands the way she wanted to, she could direct me or her dad (or anyone willing to help) as she used up a steady supply of craft materials. Most of the time, however, she was content to watch her favorite shows or read some of her favorite books. She had an incredible memory and would often re-tell stories about her favorite episodes to anyone who would listen.

Many nights, as we were falling asleep in the hospital, we'd engage in a simple ritual:

"Mommy?"

"Yes, Charlotte?"

"I want to tell you about Diego. Diego went to South America, and he found a capybara and a maned wolf."

"Yes, Charlotte. He sure did."

There would be silence for a few minutes.

"Mommy?"

"Yes, Charlotte?"

"Nemo wanted to go to school, but his dad was afraid of the sharks."

"Yes, Charlotte. Time to go to sleep."

Another long pause. Enough to think Charlotte might be asleep.

"Mommy?"

"Yes, Charlotte?"

"The Wonder Pets had to save the baby bird because he fell out of the tree."

"You are incredibly smart, Charlotte. It's time to go to sleep."

This could go on for a while.

Living in the hospital was nothing like being in our own home, but we did still manage to find some amenities that made the experience a little easier. Internet access and public Wi-Fi was a blessing from above (literally). I was able to not only keep in touch with our employees and pay bills while in the hospital, but the Internet often became a primary lifeline out of the hospital as we blogged about our experience to the world. While in the PICU, we couldn't talk on our cell phones, but we *could* send text messages. This was very handy and allowed Roger and me to converse in the wee hours of the morning or late at night without leaving her room.

In every hospital stay, there were the "good" medical professionals and the "hope to avoid" medical professionals. Notice that I didn't say "bad" or "incompetent." I don't think I ever ran into a doctor or nurse who I believed did not know what he or she was doing. All of them seemed to have the right book knowledge and smarts for the job. Some of them just seemed to be better at the personal interaction and communication piece than others.

Earlier, I mentioned Dr. Tye, Charlotte's neurosurgeon. The other key player on our team was Dr. Asadullah (Asad) Khan, our pediatric oncologist. Before we met him, we were told by the other doctors and nurses in the PICU, "Be sure to check out Dr. Khan's cowboy boots!" Of course, one of the first things I did when I met the man was look down at his feet! Dr. Khan had completed his residency in Houston at MD Anderson Cancer Center and had apparently developed an affinity for cowboy boots during his time in Texas. He was a tall, thin man with dark curly hair and a foreign accent that was both understandable and exotic all at the same time.

Doctors Tye and Khan quickly became the gold standards for medical care in our eyes. They embraced Charlotte (and us) as their patients from the very beginning and always approached Charlotte in a way that was inspirational. These were exceptional doctors who not only knew their craft but could walk into a room and assess a pediatric patient without having to poke and prod. They were never in a hurry to complete an assessment and had all kinds of tricks up their sleeve to get the information that they needed.

Their other gift was in their ability to communicate appropriately with us as parents and *listen* to our questions and concerns. They were never in a hurry to get to the next patient. They always took the time to explain what needed to be done and why. They prepared us for every step along the way. We told the doctors early on that we didn't want to tiptoe around Charlotte's needs or her situation. They honored that request with honest and simply-explained reasoning behind every procedure and medical decision along the way. It was no surprise to us that Dr. Tye and Dr. Khan quickly became Charlotte's "favorite doctors." Those were her words. She would tell everyone who asked.

> Don't be afraid to ask questions. Ask your doctors if you can communicate with them via email. Sometimes this is the easiest way for them to answer your questions. Neither one of you will feel rushed.

A herd of medical students, interns, residents, or other physicians and nurses could parade through our room. Charlotte would usually comply with their requests and occasionally engage them in cursory conversation. But if Dr. Tye or Dr. Khan entered the room, her demeanor completely changed. She positively glowed with happiness. She would get giddy and talk their ears off! It was so amusing to see the difference. She even had her own private jokes with each of them.

One of the first times Dr. Khan visited us in the hospital, Charlotte was still recovering from her second brain surgery. He walked up to the side of the bed, saying hello to Charlotte and trying to ask her a few questions. In an effort to form a friendly bond, he commented on some of her stuffed animals and Charlotte showed him a new pair of socks that looked like monkeys. These adorable socks made her toes resemble monkey puppets, complete with a little pink tongue where the monkey's mouth sat, at the tip of her toes. When Dr. Khan commented on the monkey socks, Charlotte playfully kicked her feet in his direction. Dr. Khan played back, feigning surprise and saying, "Oh my goodness! Your little monkeys scared me!" Charlotte giggled and beamed.

From that point forward, every time Charlotte saw Dr. Khan, they talked about the monkey socks. We would even make sure the monkey socks were clean so that she could wear them to clinic visits. They accompanied us on every hospital stay.

Dr. Tye and Charlotte liked to give high-fives. That was their thing. Each time he would see her, she would give him a big high-five. Although Charlotte rarely resisted going to the hospital or complained about doctor's

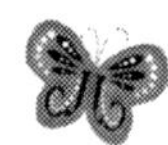

appointments, we knew that we could always brighten her day by telling her that we were probably going to see either Dr. Tye or Dr. Khan. That was something to look forward to.

Of course, anyone who works in medicine knows that it is the nurses who really do 90% of the work. These are the people on the front line who make sure the med orders go in on time, administer the medications, change dressings, clean up icky messes, communicate with the doctors, and ensure that discharge orders get completed. They page the specialists and monitor patient changes so they know when to call in the rest of the medical team. Since we spent so much time in the hospital, we quickly got to know many of the nurses and developed relationships with a few of them. We learned their names and they learned ours, or at least Charlotte's. I tried as much as possible to be a helpful mom, assisting in procedures when appropriate, changing her bedding when it was wet or soiled, getting food and drink for her on my own (when I could). You get a certain sense of familiarity at the hospital after being there for so long. Once you know the location of the icc machine or the linen closet, you kind of help yourself to a refill on water or new pillowcases-- and the nurses allow it, mainly because they are so busy with other things that you *can't* do, that it just helps the process along.

There were a few nurses along the way who were a bit annoying only because they talked too much or were a little too noisy when coming in the room at night. There were even a few who just didn't seem to have the right approach with preschool kids; we saw this most often when we ended up on the older children's area of the pediatric floor. These nurses usually just got evil nicknames from us. There was *Nurse Pee-Wee* (she reminded us of Pee- Wee Herman), *Nurse Attila,* and *Nurse Ratchet* (who made her presence known and sometimes had a matter-of-fact way about her when it came to bedside manner). There weren't many who earned nicknames, but it quickly became a funny joke between us when they did. If Roger and I were changing shifts at the hospital, we would often ask, "Who's the nurse?" and if the name offered was a nickname, we knew we were in for a fun ride.

Our one negative experience with a doctor came at MD Anderson Cancer Center in Houston, Texas. Charlotte had to see an eye doctor as one of the many regulated tests to determine baseline and monitor her progress. She had to see this doctor twice and each experience was horrible. The appointments were set for early in the morning, 8:00 a.m. or so. Each time, Roger showed up with Charlotte at the appointed time only to be kept waiting for over an hour. When the doctor finally showed, she attempted all kinds of procedures and tests on a four-year-old without approaching Charlotte *like she was a four-year-old.*

In the dimly lit room, the doctor pulled out a train on a stick with windows. Part of the train was red, another part was blue; however, there were also contrasting red and blue spots on each part of the train, near the windows.

"Can you tell me where you see the red part of the train?" the doctor would ask Charlotte unenthusiastically. Before Charlotte could even give an answer, she would ask another question or word the question differently. Even Roger was getting confused at the doctor's queries. To make matters worse, the doctor gave us no explanation as to why she was performing a particular part of the exam as the appointment progressed. She just kept going, barreling through each test saying, "OK, now just one more thing…" and then after that *one more thing* she would ask Charlotte to do something else.

Charlotte was smart enough to quickly figure out that these inane games weren't going to end any time soon and she was just *over* it. It was one of the few times that we really saw Charlotte frustrated with a medical procedure or examination that didn't involve pain. To top it all off, the doctor never seemed able to give any clear assessment of whether we needed to be concerned about her vision or not. I guess not everyone can be perfect.

The vast majority of our medical services were provided within the confines of a teaching hospital. Consequently, our lives were filled with not only doctors and nurses but interns, residents, and nursing students. I received two degrees in health-care related fields: music therapy and speech language pathology. Because of this, I understood the importance of clinicals and the opportunity to learn from *actual, live patients.* I also remember being a wide-eyed, innocent intern. (Oh, the mistakes I made.) We were informed once we came to the hospital that we should expect many students to come through our room. The reality of this experience proved interesting, to say the least.

First of all, despite any intentions on my part to remember names and titles, I instantly forgot the name of the doctor, nurse, intern, or resident to whom I was introduced when they first came into our room. If they came in a second or third time that day, I might get lucky and remember it with repetition. The pediatric floor had their own fleet of attending physicians (and residents and interns) and *then* each specialty that saw Charlotte had another set of physicians (and residents and interns).

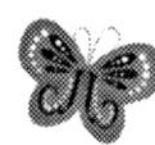

We saw professionals from the pediatric and oncology teams, but we also worked with teams from neurology, neurosurgery, infectious diseases, pediatric gynecology (yes that is a specialty), orthopedics, and dermatology. Whew!

Frequently, the students were sent in for the first round. Their job was to do the initial assessment. Then they returned with the resident or attending physician during rounds. Sometimes at this point they were accompanied by multiple doctors and students on the team so the room became rather crowded. We frequently answered the same questions multiple times to multiple people. Sometimes, when it got *really* fun, we would get to see an intern, a resident, and an attending physician all within 90 minutes but <u>not</u> at the same time. They would all ask the same questions but not always in the same way and I began to wonder (in my own bleary state of being because it was usually before 8 a.m.) if I were giving the same answers over and over again. And if we changed our story, would they mess up our daughter's treatment?

Honestly, most of the interns and residents were easy enough to deal with. The biggest challenge most interns faced was that they either A) did not want to work with pediatric patients (ever) but were required to as part of their rotation or B) they really tried and really wanted to be good at their job but just had not developed the maturity or skill for good bedside manner.

My favorite intern moments were when they would try to talk to Charlotte like she was an adult. They would ask her to rate her pain on a scale of 1-10 or 1-5. Seriously? She was three years old. Even with her intelligence, she had no concept of pain in terms of numbers. We ended up creating our own version of the pain scale. It consisted of "a little" (finger and thumb a couple inches apart), "a lot" (open hands separated by a foot or so), and "a lot-a lot" (hands wide apart). We only got that last one a few times, but it was <u>huge</u> when it happened. When Charlotte said her pain was "a lot-a lot," that was a signal to the treatment team to jump into action. She could usually describe any pain or discomfort in those terms, but of course we had to educate every medical professional on this system each time someone new came in to work with her.

Sometimes the doctors would just ask her the same old questions over and over. Charlotte had little patience for the naïve interns, and you could actually see her rolling her eyes or turning her head away when they would try to engage her in banal conversation. We began to teach her that when someone came in to ask how she was doing, she should say, "Look it up in my chart!" She mastered this task after a few days and it kept us amused!

One evening while recovering from the first two surgeries, Charlotte and I had a very sleepless night as she was fighting off a fever or some kind of infection. I knew that the interns and residents would start their rounds early so I pleaded with the nurse to let us sleep a little bit once we were able to rest. The interns were kept at bay for a while. Charlotte awoke at about 6:00 a.m. and felt really warm so I called the nurse in to take her temperature. She had a fever of 101.

When the nurse came in to check on us, she made sure I knew that she was holding the interns back. Hilariously, one intern said she needed to "see her patient and check her breathing." At this point, Charlotte was still required to be on a monitor 24/7 to track her heart rate, blood pressure, and breathing. I think the intern missed the lesson explaining that when your patient is hooked up to telemetry, you can monitor their breathing, heart rate, and pulse remotely at the nurse's station. If something goes awry, the nurses would certainly be informed via the loudly beeping machinery. The nurse calmly informed the intern that the patient was sleeping peacefully and her mom was in the room monitoring her progress. How many medical students does it take to check a patient's vitals in a 2-hour period? Apparently more than I ever imagined. Did the students think they were "cheating" if they all came in together to do their checks rather than coming separately and all finding the same information?

Probably the scariest thing about a hospital experience revolves around pain. Aside from the organic sources of pain (the disease/disorder itself), the biggest pain issue we had to deal with revolved around *needles*. When we were first admitted to the hospital, we had to fight the *dreaded needle stick* as Charlotte had multiple IVs inserted before and during her surgeries. Once we had a direction, however, we knew that a central line was part of the plan. There are two usual options for those in cancer care: a port or a Hickman. We also learned that there are advantages and disadvantages to each option.

A **port** is surgically inserted under the skin. You can have it "accessed" or "not accessed" at any given point in time. When it is being accessed, medication can go into the port and blood can be drawn out of the port. There is usually no pain involved in the process. There is some initial pain when they use a large needle to access the port, but they give some numbing cream for the skin that often helps with this. When your port is not accessed, you can swim and bathe normally and depending on its placement on your body, it may not even be visible under clothing. A port is also less prone to infection.

> ## The decision to use one type of central line or another often depends on the cancer protocol prescribed. Many types of chemotherapy (including bone marrow transplants and some *very* toxic stuff) cannot go into a port.

Hickmans, on the other hand, sit outside the skin. Like ports, they are placed in the body via surgery under general anesthesia. Once they are in, however, they are always open. They require daily flushing with heparin, an anti-coagulation drug to keep the line clear, and they cannot be submerged in water (translation: no swimming or baths). The dressing has to be changed at least weekly with a special procedure designed to minimize exposure to germs. Because of their placement and exposure, Hickmans are also more prone to infections and must be cared for carefully.

Charlotte ended up with a double lumen, or two line, Hickman and it was inserted during her second brain surgery. The nice thing about the Hickman was that although it required slightly more maintenance, we rarely had to deal with any kind of needle sticks or IVs again. All blood draws, IV fluids, and most medicine came through the central line.

After a while, Charlotte figured this out and one day she said, "A peripheral line goes in your arm or your leg. A central line goes in your chest. I love my central line." She would repeat this to the medical staff as well as to friends and family, and they were constantly amazed. If she ever seemed hesitant to work with a nurse or other medical professional, all we had to tell her was that they were going to put medicine in her line and she was A-OK with that. This also meant that Roger and I became junior nurses skilled in line care. We learned how to perform the daily heparin flushes, change the dressings, and administer medicine through the line whenever necessary. I liked to say that I was always "one procedure away from my nursing degree."

Of course, even the best attempts at medical comfort can have their share of troubles. During the second round of chemotherapy, Charlotte's central line suddenly and unexpectedly fell out of her chest. We had gone for a walk on the pediatric unit, and I was pushing Charlotte in the stroller. Upon our return to the room, I lifted her out of the stroller, holding her under her armpits. Suddenly, I saw Charlotte go in one direction and the central line fall to the floor in the other. Seeing what had happened and assessing that Charlotte didn't seem to be in any distress or pain, I paged the nurse. When she arrived and I told her what happened, I think the nurse was even more shocked than I was. Incredibly, Charlotte wasn't bleeding or in any pain. It was Saturday and because it wasn't considered an emergency procedure, we wouldn't be able to get a new central line until Monday. At that point in the chemotherapy protocol, we were simply flushing fluids through her until she could get a new medication, so we didn't exactly need the central line, but we did have to insert an IV so we could continue to push fluids. Yes, the dreaded needle sticks. I was so happy when we got that new central line!

Charlotte's other moment of terror came with the dreaded catheter. Every time she had a round of in-patient chemotherapy, they had to collect her urine for 24 hours to see if she met creatinine clearance. Basically, they needed to confirm that her kidneys were working properly in order to flush tons of toxic medication and more fluid into her system. If she had been older or more fluently continent, we would have just had her pee into a cup that would go back to the doctors, but since she was still relying on diapers, she had to be catheterized so that the urine could be collected. I can only imagine the pain and horror she felt during this process. It was so traumatizing that even months afterwards, she would occasionally say to a nurse coming into the room, "NO CATHETER!" and the nurse would need to reassure her that there would be no catheters. Not only was the insertion painful, but then she had to leave the catheter in for 24 hours and walk around with a bag attached to her hip. It was so frustrating to watch Charlotte endure this pain and discomfort and know that it was just a necessary part of the cancer treatment. Every time she urinated, she would grimace a little and you could tell that it ranked right up there as one of the most uncomfortable things she had ever experienced.

Before her brain tumor diagnosis, Charlotte had always been pretty good about taking medicine. She was a relatively healthy child before cancer entered our lives, so aside from a few rounds of antibiotics and pain relievers for the occasional fever, we had never had to worry about giving regular medicines. She took daily gummy multivitamins and she frequently told us they were "yummy." Enter the world of hospitalizations and everything changed. Although most of her medications did go through her central line, there were a few medicines she still had to take orally. The pain medications and even the oral antibiotics

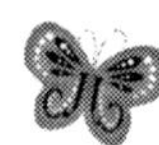

didn't present much of a problem, but the laxatives were a different story. Most of the medications they tried to give her for constipation tasted horrible and they were not easily disguised in food, milk, or juice. We tried many different options and it seemed that the more palatable alternatives didn't have any impact on her system. The few medications that did seem to work had such a horrible taste that she would gag on them, throw them up, or flat out refuse to take them. Unfortunately, this also created a trickle-down effect in which she assumed that any medication that we offered her in oral form was going to taste "yucky." Even once we found laxatives that tasted better, we had to pull out all the stops to get her to consume the necessary drugs.

Some of my favorite tricks included:

* Telling her that we were going to take the medication and pretend to put it in our mouths (a little reverse psychology). She immediately would decide then and there that she wanted it.

* Offering chocolate after the medication was consumed. This method was probably the most effective and I think this was where the Charlotte mantra "Chocolate Makes Everything Better" emerged. The trick was simple. We showed Charlotte the medicine she needed to take. She would immediately protest, so we would show her a bit of chocolate. Sometimes we would even offer to eat the chocolate ourselves if she didn't want it. This was the clincher. She would *never* let anyone eat her chocolate so she would usually relent, take her medicine, and get her chocolate in return.

* Occasionally we would even resort to sneaking some of her medicine into a glass of milk or milkshake. I was pretty sure that she was unaware of this trick until one day when we met with the nutritionist. We were concerned about her weight and her food intake. While meeting with the nutritionist looking for foods that we could get her to eat, we talked about milkshakes. I mentioned, "Maybe you can add some extra calories into it." Charlotte said, "No calories, Mommy!" She thought the "calories" were a kind of medicine that would go in the shake! The smart girl knew that we would occasionally sneak medicine into her food and milk. We promised her a chocolate milk shake with "no calories." Wouldn't we all like that?

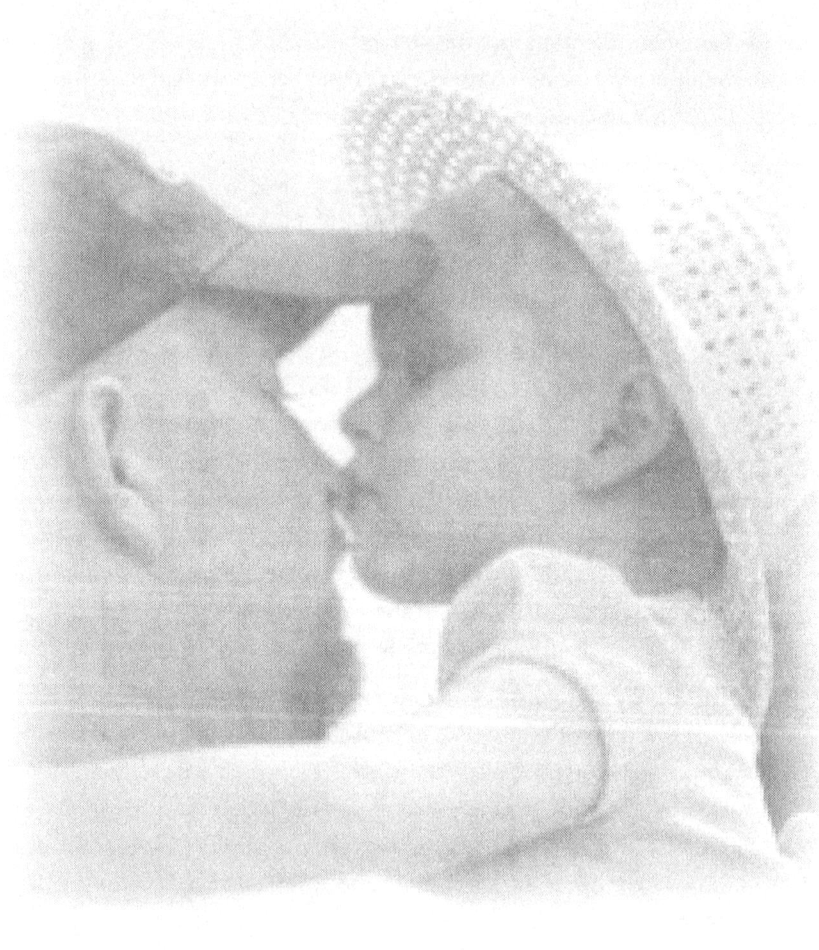

Lessons Learned from Hospital Time

"The road to Hell is paved with good intentions"
--quote attributed to St. Bernard of Clairvaux (loose translation)

The biggest learning curve I had in this entire process was not medical terminology. It was not medical procedures. It wasn't even adapting to my new schedule and daily routine. My biggest learning curve involved dealing with other people and the really ridiculous things that could (and did) come out of their mouths.

Most of the comments were well-intentioned. Actually, I think all of the comments were well-intentioned, but I'm not sure if people really *heard* the words that came out of their mouths. It ranged from the seemingly innocent ("Let me know if there's anything I can do") to the utterly ridiculous ("She has a brain tumor? Did you let her talk on a cell phone?") Yes, someone actually asked us that.

The thing is, I'm not sure if before her diagnosis I wasn't guilty of some of these proverbial foot-in-mouth situations. People don't know what to say because it's an awkward situation.

About six weeks after Charlotte died we went to visit friends that we had met in Houston. Their daughter was participating in a study with the National Institutes of Health in Washington, DC, so we made a road trip to offer our support. The visit in and of itself was bizarre. It was the first time I had set foot in a hospital since Charlotte's death. The experience was eerily familiar. As we sat there visiting with Allie and her family, I kept trying to think of things to say and I was amazed that some of the words that were on the tip of my tongue were some of the very words that had annoyed me when others said them to me. I held my tongue and realized that sometimes silence can be comforting. Sometimes people just want your presence, not advice.

Throughout the book, I'll present some of the lessons learned through our year with cancer.

Lesson #1: I don't want your snake oil

My educational background is in a field that functions based on evidence and science. I'm certified in three therapeutic and educational areas and have taken research and statistics classes at the graduate level. To that end, I was braced for the fact that we would be inundated with emails, letters, phone calls, and conversations with well-meaning people who knew "someone" who had been cured because of <u>name your miracle</u>. Some of the suggestions were actually legitimate in the form of news or journal articles; however, almost all of them were for either a different type of cancer entirely or were for something so incredibly experimental that there was no way it could be used with our daughter.

Anything that is currently in experimental trials for adults is at least 10 years away from even experimental trials with children. Further, many people don't seem to realize that just because the word "cancer" is in the title, it doesn't mean that it applies to brain tumors and, more specifically, primitive neuroectodermal tumors in kids. Every cancer is different and as we soon discovered, most cancer protocols are extremely personalized to multiple factors including: the age of the person at diagnosis, the type of cancer, and the specific location of the cancer. Furthermore, most *miracle* stories featured in news articles are anecdotal anomalies as opposed to promising evidence for most cancer patients.

The thing that always gets me about snake-oil-type claims is that we were working with a great team of extremely intelligent and accomplished physicians. We weren't being treated by the country doctor who gets paid for his services with chickens and apple pie. These were nationally recognized leaders in the oncology field who were consulting with other national leaders in the oncology field all over the country, all in world-class hospitals. If these "cures" were so successful and there was so much "evidence" that they could cure this disease, why wouldn't our doctors know about it? Were they keeping it from us as part of a grand conspiracy? Was this all because of the pharmaceutical companies? What advantage would our doctors have in hiding this information from us if it really could cure her cancer?

It was bad enough to get these types of approaches from people when we were in the midst of diagnosis, but when her condition turned terminal, it was even more difficult to hear. People would tell me that they were searching "all over the internet" for something that would cure her (Gosh, why didn't her doctors think of doing that?) or would grasp at anything that seemed remotely reasonable. I had people tell me that we needed to get second or third opinions at certain hospitals even though we were receiving treatment at MD Anderson, the biggest and best cancer hospital in the country.

We knew that her oncologists, at both hospitals, met weekly in teams with other doctors and the *Children's Oncology Group,* composed of doctors from places like MD Anderson, St. Judes, DC Childrens Hospital, National Institutes of Health, UCLA, and Boston Childrens (to name a few) were frequently conferred on these cases. We were not dealing with doctors who worked in a vacuum.

Other people told Roger or me that if we just changed her diet and had her eat an all-vegan, all-organic menu of foods, we could cure her cancer. This was *after* we were told by her doctors that there was absolutely nothing else that chemotherapy and radiation could cure. Now, I understand that there are many great foods and wonderful diets out there designed to possibly <u>prevent</u> cancer. I aim to include them in my diet on a daily basis. Furthermore, there is some evidence that for <u>adults</u>, a vegan and/or organic diet may help prevent or even reverse a course of cancer. It might even be a successful alternative to chemotherapy in some cases. It wasn't going to work for us.

The thing is, we were already grieving. We knew we would lose our child. Instead of empathizing with our loss, people wanted to find a solution, even if it meant trying to convince us that there was something out there that didn't exist. Sometimes that just poured salt on an already open wound.

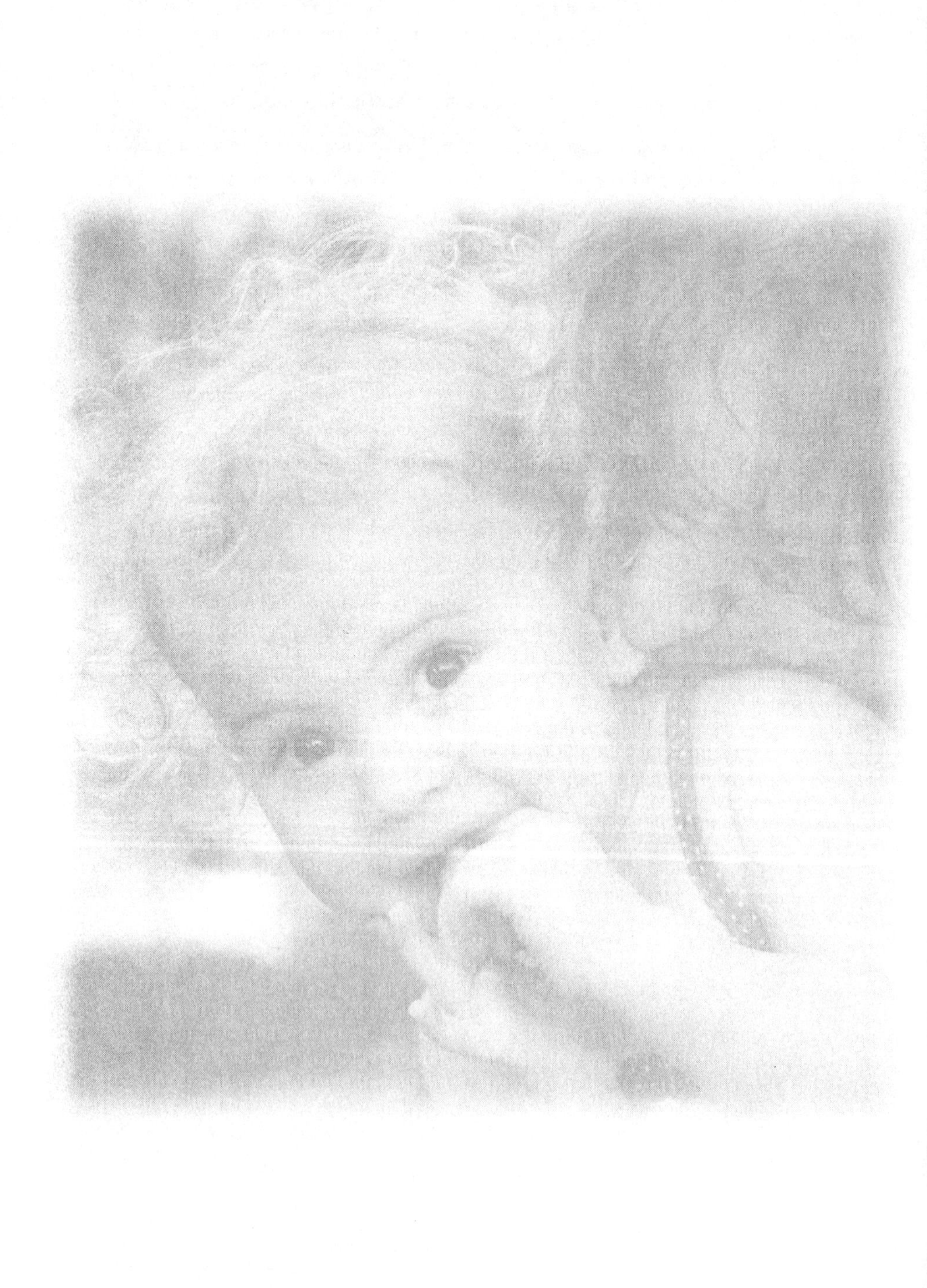

4— Course of Treatment

From the moment we heard the word *cancer*, the subsequent questions revolved around survival rates and prognosis. This was a touchy subject from the very beginning.

We didn't know what kind of tumor we were dealing with until after Charlotte's first surgery was finished and the pathology report came back. Brain tumors are rare in and of themselves (the incidence in kids is about 1 in 10,000) and then there are over 100 different *types* of brain tumors. Each one is classified by its location in the brain and the type of cells that make up the mass. Prognosis is then dictated by several more factors including the age of the patient at diagnosis, the amount of tumor that can be removed surgically, and the reactivity of the tumor cells to anti-cancer agents like medication (chemotherapy) and radiation.

Charlotte's tumor was a primitive neuroectodermal tumor or PNET. Its cause was basically unformed fetal cells that ended up in the wrong place in her body. There's usually a genetic link, although, as I mentioned, cancer didn't seem to run in our families. These tumors are extremely rare (an incidence of about 1 in 3 million) but also extremely aggressive. Because they are so rare, it is hard to narrow down accurate survival rates. About 20 years ago, survival rates were actually near zero, but thanks to advances in modern science, survival rates seem to range anywhere from about 40%-80%, depending on which study is cited. We knew going into this that those weren't great odds.

While Dr. Tye is a fabulous surgeon, he wasn't able to get the entire tumor without causing excessive brain damage due to the tumor's size and location. As he said after her first surgery, "It's a bad tumor in a bad place." This factor knocked a few points out of our favor. Very few children with PNET survive unless the tumor is fully resected with surgery: strike one.

Her age at diagnosis was also a factor. Children less than four years of age at diagnosis usually have poorer prognoses as well: strike two.

Given all that, we still had a fighting chance. So with the guidance of our oncologist, we started a cancer protocol that was the logical first step for those with PNET. The original protocol called for three rounds of induction chemotherapy (intended to keep the remaining tumor from growing), followed by three rounds of high-dose chemotherapy and stem cell transplants followed by radiation.

We began the protocol about six weeks after her second surgery. Each round was spaced about a month apart and MRI scans were scheduled every two to three months.

> If you don't feel comfortable with the options given by your doctor, ask for a second opinion at another hospital. It may be worth your time and peace of mind.

After the second round of chemotherapy, she had an MRI that yielded some inconclusive results. Usually when an MRI is completed, the radiology technicians and the doctors take an initial look, comparing the scans to any done previously as they look for significant changes. They make an initial report so that they can give worried parents and patients some kind of news about an hour after the MRI is completed. Waiting for results can be incredibly anxiety provoking. Even after this initial report, though, the radiologists and physicians will often pore over questionable scans, checking to validate their results.

At first glance, it didn't seem that the tumor had changed a great deal during the April scan, but Dr. Khan questioned some of the findings. So, he called for another MRI before we started the third round of chemo. This scan, completed on May 1, gave us the worst news to date: the tumor was not shrinking or stabilizing.

It was growing.

What this meant was that all of the toxic poison that we were injecting into Charlotte's little body wasn't working. The yucky stuff that kept her hair

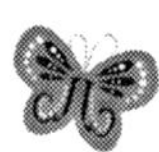

from growing and made her eyelashes fall out and put her immune system at risk for every little germ or bug was doing nothing to the monster in her head.

We were not quite at strike three, but the pitcher and the catcher were in serious conference on the mound. This is the point where we went to MD Anderson Cancer Center in Houston where some amazing doctors were working on a new treatment technique known as personalized medicine. The concept was that they would analyze Charlotte's tumor under a microscope, exposing it to different known chemotherapy agents and studying each cancer cell's life cycle. With that information, they would make a recommendation for a new treatment protocol designed just for her.

We went to Houston for the initial consultation and it was at this point that we realized the unexplored territory into which we had ventured. As we discussed survival rates and treatment protocols with her physicians, we were met with a lot of statements like, "We're not sure," or "This has been studied on a small number of patients," or "Our best guess for prognosis might be…"

Everything we were doing from this point forward was experimental. Only about a dozen patients had even attempted this personalized protocol and only one of them was a child. The results were mixed.

This was where we were and it was scary territory. What other choice did we have?

We returned from Houston and Charlotte had a third brain surgery. After viewing the most recent scans, Dr. Tye wanted another chance to remove more of the tumor, thinking that with fewer cancer cells in her brain, the new chemotherapy and radiation would have a better chance at beating up what was left. While Charlotte recovered from yet another surgery, we waited for the results from the MD Anderson research team.

We were told that the new protocol would be ready by the time Charlotte recovered from her third surgery. Given the aggressive nature of her tumor, we understood that the medical team didn't want to waste any time before starting more chemotherapy. All of the drugs we had used before were essentially "off the table," so we waited for news from the team to hear about the new plans.

The new protocol introduced a brand new set of drugs, as well as proton radiation. At the time, proton radiation was only available in about half a dozen cities in the United States. Its advantages over photon radiation include targeted, powerful radiation at the site of the tumor while minimizing both short and long term side effects. Based on all the information at our disposal, we felt it was our best chance for recovery. None of the hospitals that offered proton radiation were near Richmond. Our best bet was to return to MD Anderson in Houston where we already had a team of doctors who knew her case and had worked to develop her plan.

Charlotte turned four on July 9, 2009. Her birthdays had always been cause for celebration, but this year was a bonus beyond measure. Her party was at Romp n' Roll. We sent out an open invitation to everyone in our support circle: Bring no presents. Just show up, wear Charlotte's favorite colors (pink and/or purple), and help us celebrate. We had not just one but *three* birthday cakes donated for the occasion. It was a fun time and a great opportunity to celebrate with our supportive friends and family.

Roger and I didn't talk about it with other people, but we gave each other knowing looks all week. This could be her last birthday. I didn't want to think about it. I didn't want to say it out loud. I kept trying to push the thought from my head. I said things to myself like, *"That isn't very optimistic. You have to think positively."* The self-talk didn't work. Those thoughts were there. I knew Roger was thinking them too, but we plugged ahead: one foot in front of the other.

Right after her fourth birthday, we headed back to Texas. As luck would have it, friends in Virginia made contact with friends and family in Houston. These contacts helped us secure housing, intermittent access to a car, and other assistance. After our first weekend there, we were admitted to the Ronald McDonald House and were able to stay there for only $25 a day while Charlotte received medical treatments. The house was only two blocks from the main hospital and shuttles could take us just about anywhere we needed to go, including the proton radiation center or the grocery store. We lived in a space the size of a standard hotel room with two queen size beds, a small table, a dresser, and a bathroom. We had access to a kitchen, laundry facilities, a communal TV room, and a large play area for the kids. It wasn't home, but it would do for a few weeks.

We faced a new series of tests in preparation for radiation, including another MRI. Our oncologist at MD Anderson reported on that MRI and stated: *"The images from May 29th* [taken after Charlotte's third brain surgery] *and July 14th* [after arriving at MD Anderson] *were compared and reviewed... Some of the tumor lesions which had been left behind after the surgery became smaller during that time but there were new contrast enhancing lesions and*

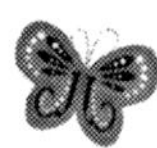

leptomeningeal disease which appears to be new. This has to be judged as a mixed response-progression."

In lay-person terms, that means that while it looked like some of the tumor left over from surgery actually got smaller, there were new tumors or lesions forming and the cancer had most definitely spread to the spinal fluid. The doctors were still confident that the proton radiation would help shrink the current tumors; however, her doctors realistically did not believe that radiation alone would be enough to fight her cancer. We were looking at a cancer that grew very quickly, very aggressively, and it was starting to spread into her spine. At this point, new drugs were added to the possible equation and we pushed forward with a mix of chemotherapy and radiation during our time in Texas.

It was right around this time that the concept of *cancer as a hurricane* seeped into my brain. Like *cancer,* a hurricane comes on strong and weaves a path of destruction. You can prepare for the battle. You can batten down the hatches. You can even move away from areas more likely to be hit by hurricanes (like Florida) to somewhere like, oh, Kansas. But then, of course, you have to worry about tornadoes and dust storms. Heck, they've even had hurricanes in Canada and England. If there's a place in the world that's not subject to natural disasters, I've yet to find it.

With some hurricanes, you have a lot of warning. You can see it coming and have plenty of time to try to minimize the effects by boarding up the windows, trimming the trees, or evacuating altogether. With other hurricanes, the storm seems to develop so suddenly, you barely have time to grab your raincoat and duck for cover. Some people choose to live in the danger zone. You can live in the tropics for years and never experience a serious hurricane. Others seem to have storms that follow their every move.

Some hurricanes are small: category one or even tropical storms. They're still dangerous and a real pain in the ass. These storms cause significant localized damage; a tree down here or there, the power goes out for a little while, school is often closed. There is preparation and clean up and all of the standard procedures. But they are far less to fear than the category five. Those powerful storms are definitely going to cause some serious destruction. Those are the ones you want to avoid. The power will be out for days or weeks at a time. Your home may be destroyed or severely damaged. You could lose everything, including your life. Because of the variable nature of these storms, sometimes when a hurricane strikes, you're still not sure (until it's passed) what category it was when it hit. It doesn't really matter. When you're in the middle of the hurricane, it's scary whether the wind is blowing at 70 or 150 mph.

And in the middle of that hurricane is an eye. The eye is deceptive. In the eye, there is no wind. No rain. No tornadoes. Everything is calm and clear. You may even hear the birds chirping. In the days before satellites and radar, people would step out of their homes during the eye of the hurricane only to be taken by surprise by the rest of the oncoming storm.

Eventually, the eye passes. Not only are you left with the rest of the storm, but sometimes the most severe, most damaging, most dangerous part of the storm is the part that follows the eye. Ironically, the most dangerous storms usually have the largest, most clearly defined eye wall.

By mid-July, we were in the eye of our own hurricane. This storm had been brewing and raging in our little family for six months. We didn't have a lot of warning, but we called out the National Guard (our incredible support system and our medical team) and they were doing the best that they could. So were we. We had been braving this storm and doing everything we could to fight it. Some days we did better than others.

Right before Charlotte's third surgery, things had been calm. We had a direction. We had a task. We hadn't spent the night in a hospital in almost three weeks (hooray). We hadn't visited the doctor's office or therapy appointments in over a week (hooray). We had actually resumed a schedule that most closely resembled our old "normal" schedule, doing things that we hadn't done in almost four months. Charlotte was happy and eating and growing and smiling and making us smile.

And yet that storm was looming on the horizon. The other side of the eye wall was getting ready to hit us and I was not sure how long the remaining storm was going to last. I was fearful of the damage that would be caused. I was fearful of the unknown. I couldn't stop thinking that the process would start all over again after her surgery. There would be risk. There would be trauma. It just came with the territory. And then there would be the long clean up. We would need to assess the damage, look towards rehab, get a new direction for cancer treatment... and the long process would begin again.

It was so difficult to look at my precious little girl and realize that while she laughed and tickled me, sang nursery rhymes, read books to herself, and talked about going to "Houston, Texas" in her adorable Southern drawl that there was this ugly, dangerous, cancerous tumor growing inside of her

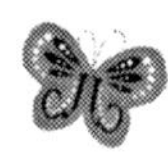

brain. That insidious thing that refused to be stopped by the traditional avenues was testing both modern science and my ability to remain optimistic.

I struggled to breathe while I sat still in the eye of the big hurricane, anticipating the storm clouds that were building again.

There is an episode of *The Simpsons* where Homer tries to gain weight and go on disability so he can work from home. In his attempt to bulk up, he goes on a super-fat diet and takes the family along with him. In a scene where Homer tries to get the kids to eat grease-upon-fat, Bart responds "Dad, my heart hurts!" and Homer replies, "Butter your bacon!"

I thought of that phrase while we entered this time in our lives. *My heart hurt,* but it wasn't from buttering the bacon. As we dug deeper into this process and I continued to realize how grave her condition was, the fact that her tumor was not dying despite the poison we put in her body, the very fact that we had to resort to experimental, aggressive, and potentially dangerous medicines to keep her alive, that made my heart hurt.

As we journeyed to Texas, the eye of the hurricane was getting ready to pass and we braced ourselves for the oncoming storm. We couldn't prepare for much because *everything*-- every step in the next part of the journey-- hung in the balance of the step that came before. Her chemo treatment would be determined by how well she responded to the surgery. Radiation would be determined by the success of the surgery and the results of the analysis. And all of the experimental stuff would hinge on how everything else played out.

In many ways, it was no wonder that we were drained from the process. For most families dealing with situations like this there is usually some sort of stabilization within the first three or four months. Families might still be in treatment, but at least they would have a plan and a terminal goal for treatments. We were still stuck in Limbo Land over six months into the process. We started out running a marathon and they changed the course.

It reminded me of the time Roger ran the Washington, DC Marathon right after the war in Iraq started (April, 2002). The company organizing the run cancelled the race at the last minute, purportedly because of terrorism and security fears. Runners, however, tend to be die-hard athletes and there was a grassroots effort to continue the race as planned. Because it was an unofficial volunteer effort, the participants had to run on the sidewalk instead of the street, there was minimal police coverage to handle traffic and they even changed the route. It was, to say the least, kind of a mess. Because of the route changes, Roger and I both got lost in the process of the run and his finishing time was less than optimal.

Would it seem ironic if I told you that he ran that race to raise money for St. Jude Children's Hospital that year?

So we were on this long course, but we didn't know if we were running a marathon, an Ironman, or a 100K race. We didn't even know where the finish line was.

Every time we got a report back on an MRI, we were knocked down a peg or two. Hope was there. Faith was there. But it was a weak candle that threatened to be dowsed at every turn. We were in the middle of the hurricane and our tiki torches were getting drenched. We prepared for the next step on the journey.

5— The New Normal

One of the first things we heard from any mental health professionals offering support immediately following Charlotte's diagnosis was, "Get ready for a new normal." Anyone who had done this before or who worked with people in crisis on a daily basis knew that our life wasn't going to be the same. Even if she was cured, fully healed, and went into remission, our lives would forever be different because of this experience.

Fortunately, we had access to counseling services through the hospital almost as soon as we were admitted, and these professionals were indispensable to our mental health. As we approached each stage of treatment, they helped allay our fears, express our anxiety and anger, focus our energy, and mitigate any frustration we had with the process. One of the first pieces of advice that I give to families that find themselves in our position is that counseling services are an important and beneficial resource.

Probably the most frustrating part of this new life was our lack of control. I like control and I am most definitely a planner. Unfortunately, I had to learn that treatment plans frequently change and hospitalizations don't always run their expected course. My child's mortality brought with it a whole host of worries and anxieties that I never thought I could endure. Many times, we had a plan in place, but the treatment cycle had to be put on hold pending scan results or blood tests. We had many doctors coordinating treatment and couldn't necessarily move forward with one thing until other particulars had been squared away.

Soon after her first surgeries and as soon as they knew the pathology of her tumor, we met with the oncologist to discuss her treatment protocol. There were all kinds of timelines that had to be followed in a particular order, but certain parts of the timeline (distribution of medications) hinged on other parts (creatinine clearance, blood test results, etc.). As they observed Charlotte's response to the treatment, they had to adjust constantly, so it was this general plan that changed almost weekly. Expected hospital stays often didn't have a set timeline and the unexpected ones *really* threw us for a loop.

Couple this with our other life stresses and it was no wonder that our sleep cycles, energy and anxiety levels, and emotions were off the charts. I was living on caffeine and adrenaline, constantly sleep deprived and anxious about what the next day, week, or month would hold. About six months into Charlotte's treatment, I finally decided that it was time to get some chemical help. Between discussions with my counselor and my doctor, we agreed that a course of antidepressants with some anxiety medication would be a good idea. It was one of the best decisions I made at the time. I'm certainly not the kind of person who thinks a pill is the solution to all of life's issues, but my body was traumatized by stress. I was in shock and my brain chemistry had changed as a result. The medications didn't make the world instantly happy, but they took the edge off so that I could at least function.

Most hospitals provide access to free or inexpensive counseling services. Use them. It is a necessary service, not a sign of weakness.

Another interesting change in my outlook revolved around my balance between working and being a mom. I never, ever wanted to be a stay-at-home mom. I always knew that I would need to go back to work after having my kids for many reasons. While the primary reason was income, the secondary reason was my sanity. I just knew that I would probably never be a great stay-at-home mom and that I needed that balance of home and work in my life. After I went back to work from my maternity leave, I never regretted it. Those first four months home with Charlotte were great but I definitely needed to go back to work. I never (OK, rarely) felt guilty or wished I stayed at home. It also helped that Roger worked part-time during Charlotte's first two years

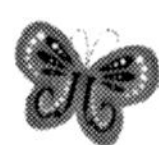

of life, so I knew that he would be home with her a great deal of the time. We didn't have to put her in full-time daycare until she was two years old.

People who know me well can tell you that I have always been Type A, motivated, efficient, and hyper-organized (maybe even to a fault). I had always been the kind of person who could be super-productive, meet deadlines, get stuff done, and stay two or three steps ahead of the game. I actually thrived on that kind of energy. My house may not have been immaculate but it was reasonably well-kept. I could work full-time with even a few part-time jobs on the side and still have time to invest my energy in church or other service organizations. Yes, that was my life before Charlotte's illness, and while it did take effort of a certain sort, I enjoyed it and it felt natural to me. That's just how I lived my life.

Fast-forward to our new situation, and I was amazed at how my perspective changed. About three months into her treatment, I wanted nothing more than to stay home and take care of my little Charlotte. I wanted to be the one who was with her, even if it meant watching that *Dora* episode for the 1000th time. I wanted to be there for all her doctor appointments and be there to watch over her.

Because of that, other things in my life took a backseat. I had trouble motivating myself to get work done. Combine this new perspective with the fatigue I was experiencing and even if I did have the motivation, I usually had neither the hours in the day nor the energy.

Piles of mail sat unopened. Emails went unanswered. Tasks on my to-do list waited until tomorrow (and the next day, and the next...). I was distracted *very* easily. Some days all I wanted to do was vegetate on the couch. I didn't recognize this new person who inhabited my body. I felt like an alien in my own skin. I knew that I should give myself a break, but I got frustrated with the lack of productivity I was experiencing. These things, in the grand scheme of it all, were relatively unimportant. And yet, I couldn't make myself truly believe it. It made me angry and I was easily frustrated. I wanted my old life and my old "self" back. I grew tired of living in crisis mode.

Repeatedly, Roger and I both heard the phrase, "I don't know how you do it" and I agreed. I had no idea. I just went from one day to the next. I put one foot in front of the other. I forced myself to get out of bed in the morning. Sometimes I cried myself to sleep. Sometimes I cried sitting at traffic lights for no apparent reason. I forced myself to go to work, to pay the bills, to get things done. Why? What other choice did I have? I couldn't let my life implode. I couldn't give up. I had to keep going for Charlotte's sake.

And yet, there were days and moments when I was genuinely, truly happy. There were moments when I laughed, smiled, found comfort, and experienced joy. They seemed fewer in number, but they were there. They were also tinged with that bittersweet taste of a *persistent sadness*.

I found myself having difficulty responding to the phrase, "How are you doing?" Compared to what? Compared to five minutes ago? Last week? Last year? My "new normal" changed so frequently that I even got sick of that terminology to describe our situation.

I gained almost 35 pounds in a year. My body was in constant anxiety mode and not only craved comfort food but didn't want to lose the pounds, even when I *did* try to eat healthfully. None of my clothes fit me anymore and it depressed me to have to shop for outfits in the plus-size department. I got frustrated that I was tired all the time and when I tried to sleep my mind ran in circles. I got frustrated at having no real schedule. I couldn't seem to figure out what we would be doing two weeks from a particular date. Forget long-range planning. That wasn't even on the table.

I had never been one to sensationalize tragedy. The "person-first language" philosophy that guided my professional life said that she was *not* a victim. *We* were not victims. She was not *suffering* from Cancer. We were not "those people" that you see on the TV news or from whose stories they make Lifetime movies. And yet there we were. This was our *New Normal.*

Roger and I each seemed to deal with the twists and turns of the year in our own way. We often shared the same perspective in the process and while we weren't always in the exact same place at the same time, we could usually understand the other person's perspective.

About three months into her diagnosis I said, "I can't do this anymore. I can't deal with everyone asking me every five minutes what to do."

"They're just trying to help," said Roger. "I think you need to give everyone a break."

"A break?" I shrieked, "I'm the one that needs the break. I don't care what we eat for dinner. Just cook something and I'll eat it. I don't care how the laundry gets finished or folded. If they're willing to do the laundry, just do it. They can't screw it up. I have enough trouble making decisions about

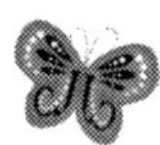

payroll and scheduling and Charlotte's health. I can't be bothered with this." I just started to cry.

Roger hugged me, letting out a big sigh and resigning himself to taking control. "OK, Dear. I'll take care of it. It's OK. We will get through this."

I would like to say there were plenty of times where the roles reversed, but I have to admit that usually I was the one getting anxious about whatever lurked on the horizon while Roger remained the calming force in most situations. It is, in part, the balance that made our relationship work.

Fortunately, we went into the *year that sucked,* as I now refer to 2009, with a strong marriage. We had been married for over ten years and had already dealt with our share of now seemingly minor crises. Sometimes we fought and sometimes we disagreed, but at the end of the day, we loved our daughter and we loved each other. I felt blessed to have someone to turn to who really seemed to understand where I was coming from.

Roger and I recognized the need to have time together as a couple. We lived together, worked together, and raised our daughter together, but like all married couples with kids, it was difficult to schedule those date nights. Now that we were stuck in the void of *Hospital Time* it became increasingly more difficult (but even more essential) to have some quality time together. We tried as often as possible to secure babysitters so that we could have dinner out, see a movie, or just go to a diner and talk. Some of the best gifts we received from friends and family were restaurant gift cards that made those date nights possible.

We spent eight weeks in Texas when Charlotte received proton radiation at MD Anderson Cancer Center in Houston. In order to keep everything in balance, we planned our eight weeks in Houston such that one of us would stay with Charlotte while the other would go back to Virginia to run the business and take care of the house. We alternated about every two weeks. One of us would fly in to Texas from Virginia on a Friday night; the other one would stay over on Saturday and fly out on Sunday to return in time for the next week's work. I think we did this a total of four times and it was crazy. Roger and I would have barely 36 hours to spend with each other, about 10 of which was spent in sleep. We made a direct and concerted effort to plan a date night each time we "traded places." We had been communicating via email and telephone all week, but it was usually for perfunctory things like business issues and Charlotte's healthcare. Most times our dates consisted simply of going out to a local restaurant where we spent hours talking and enjoying each other's company, but it was enough.

It was during this year of *New Normal* that I found such joy in the mundane and banal. I frequently wished for something *un*exciting to happen. It was a rare occasion when I could forget my troubles, relax, and go with the flow. I don't think I will ever again complain of boredom.

6— The Network

As our world crashed in on us, we experienced an interesting phenomenon that we would come to call *The Network*. While our first impulse at a time of crisis was to call on our friends and family for support, I quickly realized that retelling our medical news and updates to everyone via phone or email would soon become exhausting.

The second day that we were in the hospital, we learned of a website called CaringBridge.org that allowed us to create a free rudimentary website and blog by which we could communicate any news, updates, or events with the outside world. This became our lifeline. Within five minutes, we created a CaringBridge page for Charlotte complete with her picture and our email address in case anyone wanted to contact us directly. From there, we proceeded to tell our family and friends about the site. They told their extended family and friends. The CaringBridge page had a counter that allowed us to measure individual visits. Within a few days, the counter was in the thousands. People left messages on our guestbook and we received notes from not only friends and family but complete strangers who had learned of us through prayer circles and acquaintances. Within three months, we had posted over 100,000 visits and over our time on CaringBridge (almost a year), there were at least 3000 unique visitors to the site. By the time of her second surgery, after only two weeks in the hospital, we realized that there were individuals in every continent (except maybe Antarctica) praying for our daughter and following our story.

CaringBridge was perfect for us. We were able to provide updates to *The Network* on Charlotte's ongoing medical condition and this kept us from having to repeat stories multiple times. Roger and I shared in the writing, frequently alternating posts. When we bumped into friends and acquaintances outside of the hospital, they didn't have to say, "How is Charlotte?" but rather started the conversation based on what had been posted in our last update. Roger and I both found it easy to be honest and open about our feelings throughout the process and the writing became a therapeutic outlet.

CaringBridge also served as a focal point for energizing *The Network*. When we found it necessary to organize fundraisers, locate child care, get help with meals, or other family needs, we would post it on CaringBridge. Within minutes of a post, I would get emails or calls from people willing to help in any way. I would mention a yearning for chocolate, and freshly baked cookies would show up at the hospital. Roger would share that Charlotte's favorite TV show of the moment was *Dora the Explorer,* and we would get three new videos or a brand-new coloring book delivered to our house. It was like Aladdin's magic lamp!

We found other people who had pages on CaringBridge. They would sometimes find us and post messages in our guestbook. This led us to more families who were experiencing the same thing or were on similar journeys. We began subscribing to their CaringBridge pages, following their stories and supporting them as well. In a similar way, when we met others at the hospital enduring treatment for a chronic illness, we directed them to CaringBridge or asked if they had their own blog or website. CaringBridge was like Facebook for sick people.

> The Internet can be very helpful. Use social media to communicate when you are comfortable, even if it's just to tell people that you don't want to talk.

In fact, that became another amazing tool for launching *The Network,* as well. Roger began using Facebook during his college professor days, and I begrudgingly joined up about three months before Charlotte's diagnosis at the prodding of some high school friends.

I quickly became addicted.

Social media tools like Facebook were great for reconnecting with friends from high school and college. Little did I know what kind of role these networks would play as we entered this phase of our lives. I think my first post upon realizing Charlotte's diagnosis was, "*I truly believe that God doesn't*

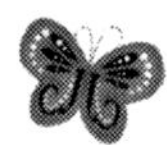

give us more than we can handle, but I sure am feeling tested." Immediately the queries began. Friends wondered what was going on and as we shared the news, the word spread around the Facebook community. An acquaintance in our town started a fan page for Charlotte titled *Get Well Charlotte Reynolds.* I didn't even know about it until another friend said, "I heard Charlotte has her own Facebook page!"

We used the CaringBridge and Facebook pages to gather support and spread news about fundraisers and events. We received cards, gifts, and good wishes from complete strangers. A few months after her diagnosis, we began receiving notes in the mail from the Secret Angel Stitchers. This is a group of women from all around the world that create machine-stitched ornaments and trinkets, usually bears, angels, hearts, etc., and mail them anonymously with a sweet note or a prayer. We would receive one or two a day for over a month! The pieces were delicate and beautiful, and we would marvel at each homemade work of art.

Other gifts from charitable organizations found their way into our home. The Princess Alexa Foundation sent us two full princess outfits, complete with gloves, tiaras, and jewelry. Charitable organizations sent us cute hats when Charlotte's hair fell out. We received prayer shawls from church groups and individuals.

Gifts came in from everywhere for Charlotte and for us: videos, games, books, stuffed animals of every kind, clothes, hats, blankets, coloring books (and any other craft goodie you could imagine), balloons, cards, jewelry, snacks. It was actually overwhelming. Gifts were delivered to the hospital and to our house. We finally had to blatantly ask people to not bring gifts to the hospital because we were running out of space in her room.

The families from her preschool got together and bought us a standalone freezer to store all the meals that people brought for us. Others gave us gift cards to restaurants and the grocery store, Starbucks coffee cards (manna from heaven), and items with which to pamper ourselves like lotions, soaps, and aromatherapy.

We became local celebrities… for all the wrong reasons. Only a week or so after her diagnosis, Todd, one of the fathers in Roger's Dads Group, told me that he was at the gym talking to someone about us and our situation. Another friend of ours who didn't know Todd overheard the story and said, "Charlotte? Charlotte Reynolds? I know her!" It was unbelievable. We made the local paper a few times with news of our story or upcoming fundraisers.

The reporter who writes the weekly news for our tiny town of Ashland mentioned our story and charted our progress frequently during the year. At one point, I think Charlotte was the most famous four-year-old in Richmond.

There came a point about three months into the process where we realized that we might need some financial assistance to ease our burden. Fortunately, most of our medical expenses were currently covered by our health insurance, but even though the *actual* cost for one of her surgeries was around $20,000 and insurance paid a large part, we received a bill for about $2,000 to cover additional medical expenses. That was from one surgery. We didn't have a lot of savings just "lying around." The larger concern came when we faced the possibility of out-of-network expenses if we needed to pursue the stem cell transplants at our local hospital (instead of going to an in-network hospital over three hours away). These out-of-pocket expenses were estimated to be about $30,000 per round of chemotherapy.

When it came to money, I didn't really worry about the medical expenses. They were definitely real and there was certainly a potential for the costs associated with her care to spin out of control; however, I knew that in a worst-case scenario, we would set up payment plans with each hospital and pay what we could, when we could, even if it took decades to pay the money back. One of my bigger concerns was helping us make ends meet with our personal expenses associated with travel, food, and more while we jumped from hospital to hospital, took time away from work, and altered our lifestyle in order to care for our daughter. We were already pretty much living from paycheck to paycheck. Strike that. Because of the challenges with our business and the impact of the recession, we often relied on borrowed money to make up for shortfalls at the end of a month. I realized quickly that we might need some financial assistance.

> ### Find a few friends who might be interested in organizing the fundraisers so that you can focus on caring for your child.

People asked what they could do to help so we set up an account in Charlotte's name at a local bank and shared the information with our network of friends. We made it clear that, because we were not an official nonprofit organization, donations to our family couldn't be considered tax-deductible;

however, we promised to use the donated funds exclusively for Charlotte's medical expenses or our travel expenses related to her care.

The Network mobilized for a variety of very successful fundraisers. One person had the idea to create and sell plastic bracelets (similar to the yellow Lance Armstrong *LiveStrong*) as a visible sign of support for our cause. Our bracelets were pink and said *Prayers for Charlotte*. Family, friends, and strangers from all across the country purchased the bracelets and it became an easy fundraising endeavor.

Our first major fundraising event was a Head Shaving Party. We knew that Charlotte would lose her hair due to the chemotherapy and we saw the Head Shaving Party as a fun way to help her deal with this process. In the end, I don't think Charlotte's hair falling out was a big deal to her. It started falling out very quickly after her first round of chemotherapy and we replaced the hair with fun hats and other things to distract her. Charlotte didn't seem to mind. I really missed those golden curls, but after a while, it was hard for me to picture her with hair. She just became my favorite "bald chick."

We had about ten friends, including two kids, who volunteered their tresses for the cause. Each person collected pledges before and during the event and we had prizes donated for those that collected the most money. We held the party at Romp n' Roll and while all of Charlotte's peers played in the gym, the brave souls had their heads shaved in our art room. The event raised over $5000! It was an amazing sign of support for our cause.

Similar events followed throughout the year including a bake sale, a home-business bazaar, and a burrito-eating contest sponsored by Qdoba, a Mexican restaurant chain. The money raised through these events helped cover our out-of-pocket medical expenses, travel expenses, and other incidentals we encountered throughout the year due to the frequent trips in and out of the hospital. While most of the events were held close to home, our families held their own yard sales, bake sales, and bazaars in Colorado, New Mexico, Tennessee, and Florida. These signs of support not only helped with our financial stress but also bolstered our spirits as a tangible sign of the spiritual support we were receiving from *The Network*.

The power of *The Network* was evident in other ways as well. In May, our friend Megan was nominated for a contest sponsored by a new local website called Richmond Mom. Megan began her cancer journey only a few months before we did as she was diagnosed with breast cancer the day before Thanksgiving, 2008. She was going through treatments alongside Charlotte.

They even lost their hair the same week! The contest in which Megan was participating had friends nominate *great moms* in the Richmond area to win a package full of fabulous prizes, just in time for Mothers Day. As a cancer warrior, special needs advocate, and mom of two young kids, Megan certainly fit the bill. The winner would be determined by internet vote so we did everything we could to help rally *The Network* for votes of support. We announced the contest on CaringBridge and on our Facebook sites. When Megan won the Great Richmond Mom contest we were thrilled for her.

One month later, the website sponsored a new contest for Father's Day. I nominated Roger, but I wasn't alone. He actually got three nominations. We fired up *The Network* again and we were overjoyed when Roger won. He got a year's worth of Chick-Fil-A (that's like gold in our house) as well as some other fabulous prizes and an awards ceremony.

Finally, September rolled around and Richmond Mom had another contest to offer. This time it was a Mommy Makeover. Unbeknownst to me, Roger submitted a nomination on my behalf. I almost didn't accept the nomination because of some impending events on my calendar. Then I figured that I might as well enter the contest just to see what would happen. Who couldn't use a makeover in my situation? So we activated *The Network* again. This contest selected three finalists, all of whom would receive a salon experience with a new hairstyle and makeup as well as a brand-new outfit from a local clothing retailer. It was like one of those reality makeover shows. The overall winner received another fabulous prize package revealed at an elegant wine reception the evening of our makeover. *The Network* did their job and I not only made it into the final three for a makeover experience, but I actually won the contest.

Needless to say, Kate Hall, the founder of the Richmond Mom website, was amazed by our story. She couldn't believe that Roger and I had won our respective contests and helped Megan win hers. We promised that we wouldn't win any more contests for the rest of the year.

One of the most surprising parts of *The Network* was our Romp n' Roll community. The day of her diagnosis, our employees kicked into full gear and covered whatever they could for us. At the time, Roger and I were teaching the majority of classes and covering many shifts. This was our full time job and all of our other employees worked part-time. Many on our staff were college students. It didn't seem to matter, though. During the next year, we were not able to work anywhere close to full-time and our staff always did

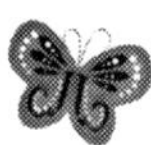

whatever was necessary to cover classes and parties. During the entire year, we never had to cancel a class or party. I always managed to file payroll and other bills on time. Amazingly, we stayed in business even in the midst of a recession and a health crisis.

The week that she went into the hospital, our manager put up a picture of Charlotte in the lobby with a sign saying "Please Pray for Charlotte." She also posted links to the CaringBridge site for anyone who was interested. Charlotte had always been a fixture at the store, hanging out with us after preschool and frequently participating in the classes that she loved, so most of our customers knew her. Almost immediately, cards and gifts came in to the store and the hospital from our customers. During the year, some of our customers would bring our family meals, coffee, and other goodies. We had one customer who would just give us $20 every time she came in (every few weeks) and told us to "go out to lunch or something" with the money. A week after Charlotte's diagnosis, I found an anonymous envelope on the dashboard of my car with the words "from a Romp n' Roll mom that cares" written on the front. The envelope contained $40. The store became a central hub for fundraisers and a drop-off point for meals. Our customers offered to cover shifts or volunteer their time in any way that was needed.

It was amazing. Roger and I had always said that as business owners one of our main goals (aside from making money) was to create a sense of community in our store. We wanted it to be more than just a place where people brought their kids to play. It was through Charlotte's illness that I realized our mission as business owners had been achieved.

One final group in *The Network* that must be mentioned is our family. Living in Virginia, we were miles away from the majority of our close and extended family units. At the time, most of Roger's family lived in Colorado and New Mexico. Almost all of my family lived in Florida. Roger's dad lived in Tennessee. Aside from one cousin who lived across town and my brother who lived next door to us, the majority of our relatives lived at least a day's drive away. This didn't seem to matter, though, because our family mobilized to support us in any way they could. Those who could visit scheduled to stay with us for a week or two at a time and provided support, alternating weeks with one another. They took time from their jobs and families to field phone calls, stay with Charlotte so that Roger and I could work, make meals, do the laundry, clean the house, and provide a much-needed emotional crutch. There were very few times during the year that we didn't have some family staying with us. Our families also supported us from a distance by sending care packages and offering an ear when the stress necessitated some emotional venting.

When people remarked at how well Roger and I balanced everything in our lives during this time, I often said that *The Network* was what made it all possible. While we didn't always feel it at the time, Roger and I did have the strength to weather our adversity, but we were also bolstered by *The Network* which was made up of hundreds (thousands?) of people who cared about us. They would do anything for us. They picked us up when we were down. It was alright to stumble and fall because we knew we would be caught. At the very least it would be a soft landing.

Lesson #2: Just do it!

I love the maxim *It's easier to ask for forgiveness than permission.* I think the corollary to this in the cancer world is: Don't say *If there's anything I can do to help...* Just find a problem and fix it! Almost everyone we would run into would use the former phrase. It's kind of like when you ask, "How ya doin'?" in casual conversation but you're not really expecting a reply. You're not expecting the person to say, "Well, I'm actually having a pretty bad day. How the heck are you?" It's just something you say to fill up the space.

We really did need help with many things, but we were often so emotionally and physically tired that we didn't have the energy to direct anyone. The big need was for people to see a gap and to fill it. I was appreciative for all the favors that people did for us, but I was *most* appreciative when I didn't have to ask. We found this in big favors like getting an electrician to come to the store and install some new lights for us or having friends clean our house after we had been away for a weekend. We also found this in small favors like gift cards for Starbucks or one of our favorite restaurants waiting for us in an envelope, dinner brought to our door each night, or small bags of 'goodies' left on our front door (cookies, coffee, homemade hummus you name it).

One of the most interesting observations I made in the process revolved around the phrase, "Our thoughts and prayers are with you." If I had a nickel for every time I heard that phrase or saw it written in a card or email, I could finance a new wing of the hospital. Individually, the phrase carried no weight. It was just something to say to fill the void when no other words seemed right. On the other hand, when I would read comments on our blog or Facebook pages or look at the piles and piles of cards in Charlotte's room that had been sent from all over the world, I felt the impact of that phrase. *Our thoughts and prayers are with you.* Can you imagine? There were hundreds—no thousands of individuals thinking of us, sending positive vibes, and praying for us. It created an energy force that was strong and comforting at the same time. It was like a huge, soft blanket on which we could break the freefall that had become our lives. And for that I continue to be grateful.

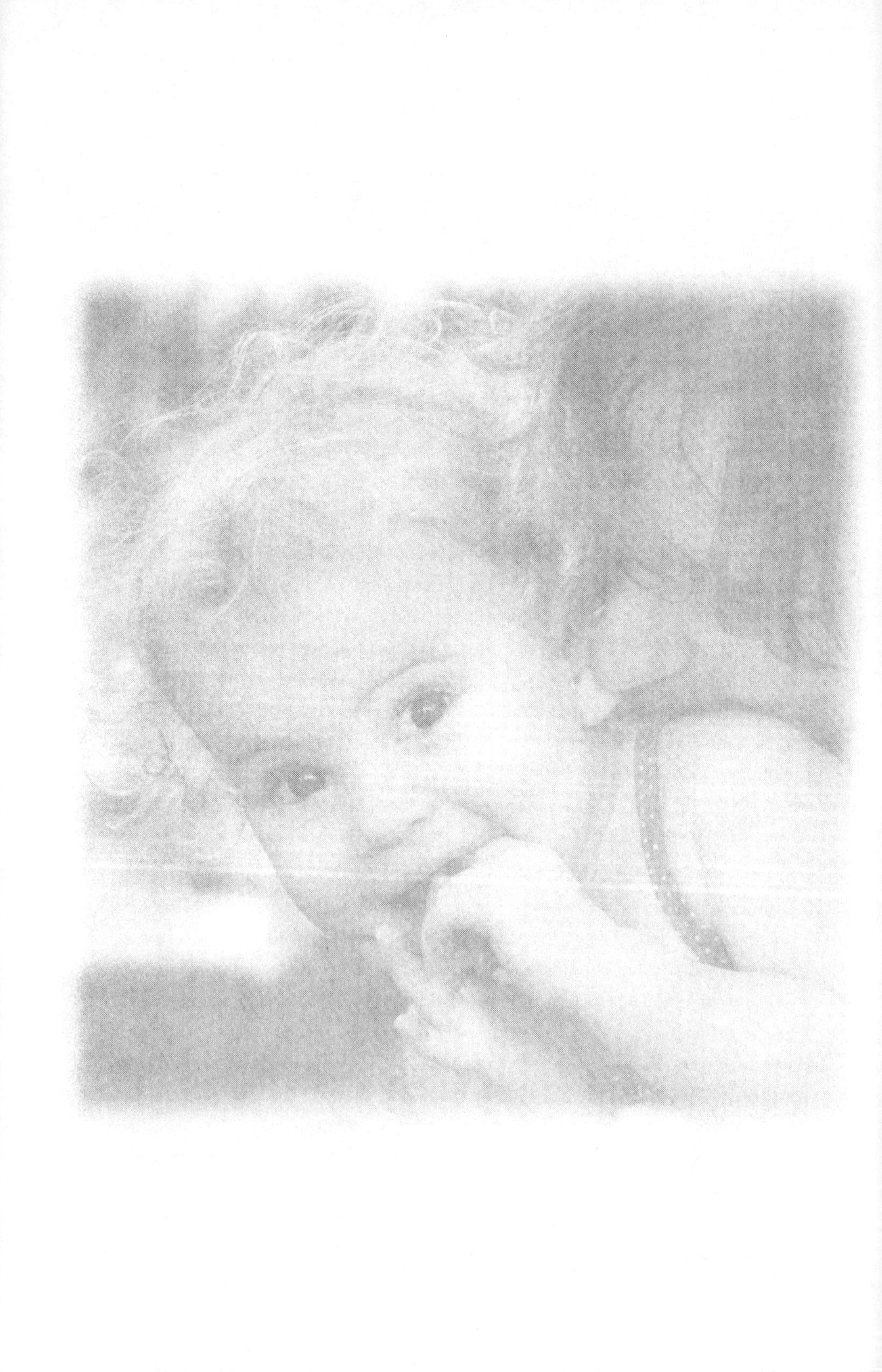

7— Circles of Faith

"So in Christ we who are many form one body, and each member belongs to all the others" — Romans 12:5

My father died when I was eight years old and the support that my mother, brother, and I received from our church family was incomparable. It was my first exposure to the true meaning of the phrase *Community of Believers*. I've always found a sense of comfort in a church home. To me, it's about more than the dogma of religion. You can practice your beliefs anywhere, but the church becomes an extension of your family wherever you go. In my adult life, I was rather selective about the churches I joined and searched for that sense of community wherever we lived.

I was raised in the Presbyterian tradition, but experienced a sampling of every type of Christian denomination while growing up. As an adult, I found the most comfort and spiritual fulfillment in the Episcopal tradition.

We lived in Fredericksburg, VA from 2001-2003. This was the first time since college that Roger and I felt "settled" and ready to commit to a congregation. We weren't in school or moving every year or two. It was also the first time since leaving high school that I felt ready in my spiritual journey to make a commitment to a church congregation. In our search, we found a fabulous Episcopal community at Trinity Church, a fairly large congregation, adjacent to a college campus, with a variety of opportunities for active ministry. Even Roger, not usually a *religious* person in the traditional sense, enjoyed his involvement with the congregation there. We loved the church so much that we kept our membership active even after we moved almost 45 minutes away. Charlotte was baptized in that church and it was a very difficult move to find a church closer to our Ashland home in 2007.

When the time came to find another congregation, I was, again, very selective. We took it slow, visiting places closer to our house and spending almost a year going back and forth between about half a dozen Episcopal churches before settling at St. James the Less. We had been members there for a little over two years when Charlotte was diagnosed. Ed Tracy, our pastor, was with us through every step of Charlotte's journey, making frequent visits to the hospital and our home when needed. The church posted links to our CaringBridge site on their website and our church family surrounded us with emotional, spiritual, and tangible support.

Our families' churches played a huge role in our journey as well. My parents were involved in at least two congregations in Florida that learned of our story. One congregation put together a fundraiser that netted over $5000. We also received cards, gifts, and letters from members of this church. These were people who had never met Charlotte or me, but they cared enough about my parents to support them in their grief process as well. Roger's father had connections with his church in Tennessee that supported us similarly.

I was continually touched by the kindness, thoughtfulness and poignancy of Charlotte's peers. Children are so spiritually minded—I think it is just a natural state of being for them. I'm not even talking about religion, per se, but a heightened sense of that greater Spirit that envelops us, guides us, and protects us. It hearkens to mind the Biblical allusions where we are called to come to God "like a child." Between Charlotte's peers at church and school and our customers at Romp n' Roll, we were surrounded by children on a daily basis. It was natural that curiosity would often lead the children to ask questions. Sometimes parents would apologize or try to keep the kids from asking these difficult questions. Roger and I didn't mind and we always tried to answer honestly and at their level of understanding.

"Why is she sick? Is she going to get better?" one would ask. "Well, she has a tumor in her head. The tumor is not supposed to be there so the doctors are giving her medicine or doing surgery to try to get it out. They are doing the best they can to make her better," I would say.

"Why doesn't she have any hair?" asked a little boy at the mall who looked to be about six years old. Roger responded, "She has a disease called cancer. The medicine they give her to fight the cancer makes some other things in her body stop growing for a little while. When her hair stopped growing, it fell out."

"Is it going to come back?" he continued to query.

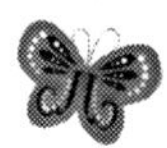

"Yes. Eventually her hair will grow back. It might look a little different, but her hair will start to grow again after the medicine is finished working in her body," Roger explained.

"Why does she have that brace on her leg?" asked one of Charlotte's peers as they played at Romp n' Roll. "Charlotte had to have a surgery and the surgery made her arm and her leg weak on one side. She wears the brace and does special exercises to get stronger," I explained as we moved around the equipment in the gym.

After Charlotte died, sometimes her friends would come up to us and ask us other questions. "Did Charlotte go away?" "Where did Charlotte go?" Interestingly, though, many times instead of questions, the children talked about Charlotte in declarative statements, much like understood tenets of faith. "Charlotte went to be with the angels." "I drew this picture for Charlotte and for you. I miss her." "Charlotte turned into a butterfly and flew away." "I sent my balloon up to visit Charlotte. I hope she can see it." I have no doubt that these children understood what it meant to lose a friend despite their youth. The thing that amazed me was the wide-eyed but matter-of-fact innocence with which these young sages approached the concept of life and death. They knew it was a time to be sad, but they didn't seem to be scared or angry. The children seemed to approach Charlotte's loss with faith and grace.

Children trust inherently that their caretakers will provide for their every need. They trust in the wisdom of their parents as omniscient beings (at least until they become tweenagers) and they instinctively know that their parents will protect them in times of danger. I think as grown-ups, it is so much easier to let the cynicism and hard realities of life create negative energy. We forget to trust God, especially when it matters most. Typically children, on the other hand, are just naturally positive.

As Charlotte's days grew shorter, our spiritual havens supported us in less tangible, but still powerful ways. While we had received cards and even a few gifts and visits from our church home in Fredericksburg, we hadn't seen many of the members of the congregation throughout the year. When Charlotte received the terminal diagnosis, I called our pastor there and asked if we could have a simple prayer service one evening. We found a suitable Saturday and journeyed to Fredericksburg for the service. The church was decorated with pink and purple balloons. We had a beautiful, simple evening prayer service called Compline, and then had an opportunity for fellowship in the church hall. For those who hadn't had the opportunity to visit Charlotte in the hospital or any other time during the last year, it was a beautiful way for them to say goodbye.

As much as I relied on our church family during that year and the time that followed Charlotte's death, it is important to acknowledge, however, that sometimes church just wasn't comfortable. I tried to attend services as regularly as possible, but even if I was home on a Sunday, I was often too emotionally or physically spent to make it to church. Other times, I would make it to church, but would get so overwhelmed by the good intentions of "support" that I almost felt smothered. Some of those well-meaning phrases like "I know God will heal her" would creep into the conversations and it would just be too much. Sometimes I just didn't want to answer the question "How are *you* doing?" one more time. Sometimes I just wanted to be alone with God. So I was. It was interesting to me because I never imagined that this would be my reaction, given my previous spiritual experiences within the church.

After Charlotte passed away, I drifted further from the church for a while. There were many reasons. Some were logistical. Work responsibilities had me covering shifts on Sundays. Sometimes I didn't have to work on Sunday, but it was my one true day of rest and my only day to sleep in, relax, or catch up on the week's chaos. I just didn't have the energy for church.

The main reason for my absence, though, was that the few times that I ventured to church soon after Charlotte's passing, the experiences were incredibly uncomfortable. It had nothing to do with the people there. Everyone was kind and supportive and seemed genuinely happy to see me. I just saw Charlotte *everywhere* and it was painful.

As I sat in the pew one Sunday morning, I realized that I just couldn't keep coming to church. There were many weeks that I left church on the verge of tears or I cried in my car after leaving the service. This week, I barely made it into the parking lot. My stomach started churning. I felt my pace quicken. My heart ached. Tears leaked out before I had turned off the ignition in my car. I took a deep breath and composed myself. I'd be OK once I got into church. I'd be fine once I saw familiar, supportive faces in the congregation. I was wrong.

I made a right turn instead of a left as I made my way from the parking lot into the church itself. Why did I go this way? I realized I was avoiding the walk past the nursery. I couldn't look at those other kids playing where

 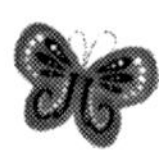

she had played. I couldn't bear the sight of Charlotte's friends sharing songs, books, cookies, and apple juice without her.

I found a seat in the pew. I tried to absorb my thoughts in the ritual of the service. I listened to the sermon. I participated in the scripture readings. I could feel myself becoming calmer. I was OK. I was comfortable. I was getting in touch with that inner peace that church could provide.

Then it was time for communion. It all came flooding back: the anxiety, the tears, the memories of taking Charlotte's hand as we walked up the aisle to the communion rail. She would put her small hands out for the communion wafer. She would receive her blessing and then we would pray the simple prayer that I had taught her: "Thank you, God, for all my blessings." I couldn't do it. If church was going to fill me with anxiety from week to week, I couldn't make it a part of my life anymore. Church was supposed to make me feel better… not worse. After that Sunday, I avoided my "home" church completely. Roger actually found a job singing with a church on the other side of town. I occasionally attended a service, usually around the holidays, making an appearance with the choir to provide an extra voice. It was easier to be in an unfamiliar setting, but I found those feelings of anxiety slowly creeping in each time a familiar ritual evoked strong memories of Charlotte.

I found it strange that church would cause this reaction while working at Romp n' Roll, surrounded by kids on a daily basis, did not evoke this kind of feeling. Somehow my mind was able to separate the working aspect of my life from my personal and leisure time. There were plenty of times where I had been at Romp n' Roll without Charlotte but there was rarely a time where Charlotte and I did not share an experience at church. I saw her peers continuing to participate in these activities and felt her absence much more clearly at church than anywhere else in my life.

My heart is still in the church and my life still embraces these concepts of spirituality, but I find more comfort these days in my personal spirituality than in a shared sense of spiritual community.

Roger's spirituality, while strong in its own sense, can be a little on the unconventional side. My mother likes to refer to Roger endearingly as *her pagan son-in-law*. While he has never rejected formal religion per se, he is not inclined to participate in formal worship on his own and doesn't take communion. That being said, Roger has an exceptional spirituality to him. On the surface it may seem that our religious views differ, but I would argue that they are very much alike in many ways. I think that is one of the reasons why throughout this process we frequently viewed our situation from the same vantage point spiritually. One of Roger's blog posts, from early November 2009, just following her terminal diagnosis, really sums it all up:

I am thoroughly convinced that things happen for a reason. There has to be something holding the universe together; otherwise, according to chaos theory and quantum physics, there's no reason why we shouldn't all suddenly turn into random objects like ashtrays and lawn mowers, or have VWs growing out of our heads at strange angles. We have no idea the reasons but they are there. My latest mantra is: Don't try to find the reason in the darkness of the moment. The reason will show itself eventually. Right now there is no reason. It's my version of faith.

That doesn't mean we're sitting back and just letting things happen. Our doctors are reaching out, discussing Charlotte's case with other colleagues and we will be seeking out alternative therapies like acupressure and chiropractic if for no other purpose than to manage any pain. The absolute main goal is for Charlotte to be as comfortable and functional as long as possible.

This brings me back to my discussion on spirituality and the word of the day: Grace. It's a word that has been floating around in my brain for quite a while and I'm still digesting it but I feel I'm finally starting to get the slightest glimpse of its true meaning. Kung Fu *is one of my favorite TV shows of all time, full of little tidbits of wisdom including one I still use. "When a man finds his true path, Heaven is gentle." That, very loosely, is what grace means to me. It's that Michael Brecker concert back in 1988 on the University of Miami patio that reached deep inside me and showed me what power music could wield. It's that bartender at the Invershin Inn in Scotland who pulled out a guitar and reignited my passion for music. It's the "Home" feeling I get when I'm teaching at Romp n' Roll. It's the conviction I feel that Charlotte came here intentionally; that she chose us to be her parents because of some purpose way beyond our ability to comprehend. It's asking the network for a pony ride for Charlotte and getting 50 offers in an hour.*

Here's something else... In Robert Schimmel's book, Cancer on $5 a Day (Chemo Not Included), *he mentioned his son who had died from cancer some years before. He said his son was an old soul and that he believes they had known each other before. It's easy for me to imagine that for Charlotte considering how easily she learns things and the amazingly deep connection she and I share but the one thing keeping me from truly believing that is the pure wonder with which she seems to view everything. Like a very young soul.*

So my take on it is that she is a "wondering/wandering" soul who came here this time to learn and to touch peoples' hearts. And she has done both extremely

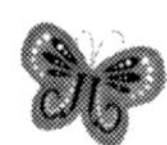

well. I know I'm biased and (trying not to sound trite) that ALL children are special but I look at all the people Charlotte has touched, even those who have only heard about her or just seen a photograph, and I can't help but be convinced that she has something extra special about her. How many of you fell in love with her the moment you saw or met her? It's more than just chemical or visual. She has SOMETHING about her and I can't tell you how privileged (full of grace?) I feel to have been allowed to be her parent; to watch her "collect" people's hearts and see that special something in action.

I've got to agree with him on so many levels. Grace… Karma… Life Force. Call it what you will, but there is a spiritual force in this world. It keeps the sun rising, the tides rolling, and our hearts beating. It is what helps us get out of bed each day. It gives us purpose. It gives us a sense of community. It allows us to heal when our hearts have been wounded.

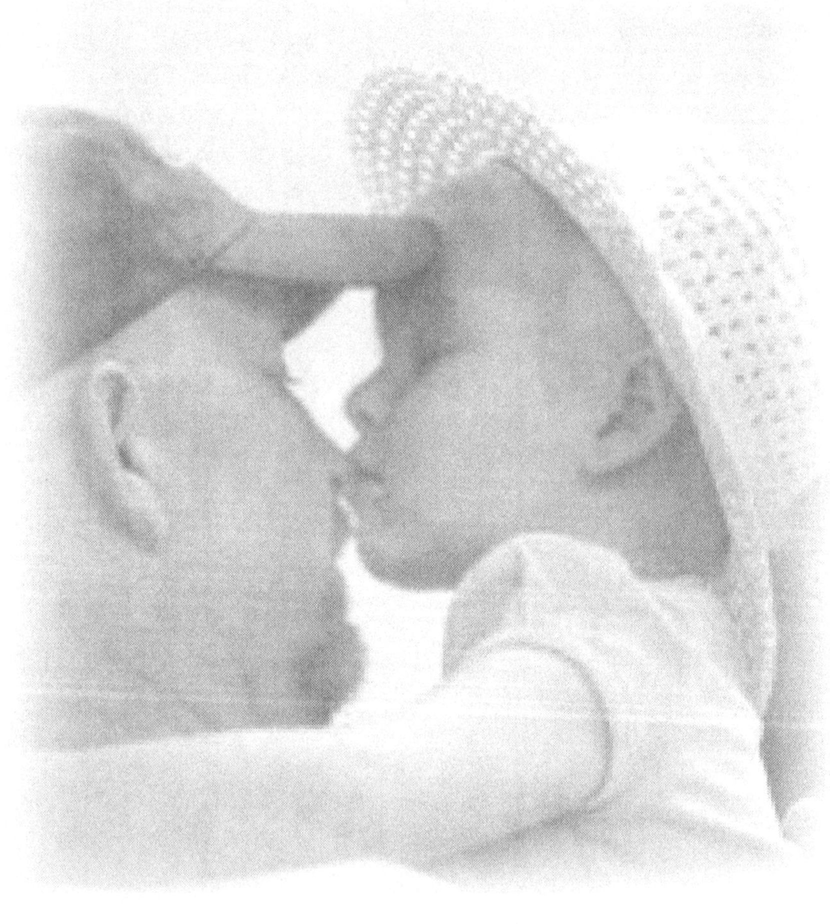

Lesson #3: If you're going to use religion, tread with caution

My faith is extremely important to me and helped me through this process. That being said, there are some people (I will politely refer to them as *zealots)* who can bring some interesting and not necessarily comforting perspectives to the process. Comments such as, "God will heal her if we believe enough," or saying "I know that we will get a miracle," even after her diagnosis was deemed terminal by the doctors, were not in any way comforting to me.

Sometimes they even let these *zealots* volunteer their time at the hospital. One Sunday while Charlotte was getting her second round of chemotherapy, we went to "Sunday School" on the hospital floor. Charlotte made a butterfly and heard a few stories. The event was attended by about half a dozen kids, all but one of which were between the ages of 1 and 5. The lesson started out innocuously, but it quickly devolved into a lesson in heaven-and hell-theology with a bunch of preschoolers. I have no idea what church this pastor was from or what her religious dogma entailed specifically, but we were treated to a good ol' Bible tract and the concept that "There are only two places to go when you die: Heaven or to live in the fiery pit." This is *an exact quote* of what the woman said to these kids.

The most ridiculous part to me was that someone would even talk about Heaven and Hell theology with a bunch of sick kids and their parents. What about Grace? What about Healing? What about the Peace that Passes all Understanding? How about just a rousing chorus of "Jesus Loves Me"? That might make for better hospital conversation.

It's also important to remember that not everyone shares the same beliefs in life, death, heaven, or an afterlife. Some parents take serious offense to the idea of their child as "an angel in heaven" because that is not how they imagine them to be after death. Further, the phrase *"I know that she is in a better place"* is particularly bothersome. In my mind, there was and is no better place for Charlotte to be than *with me.* Here on earth. It is not necessarily comforting, even if I believe in Heaven and the afterlife, to think that she is somewhere else. In fact, sometimes the use of that phrase is extremely painful to the person who is grieving.

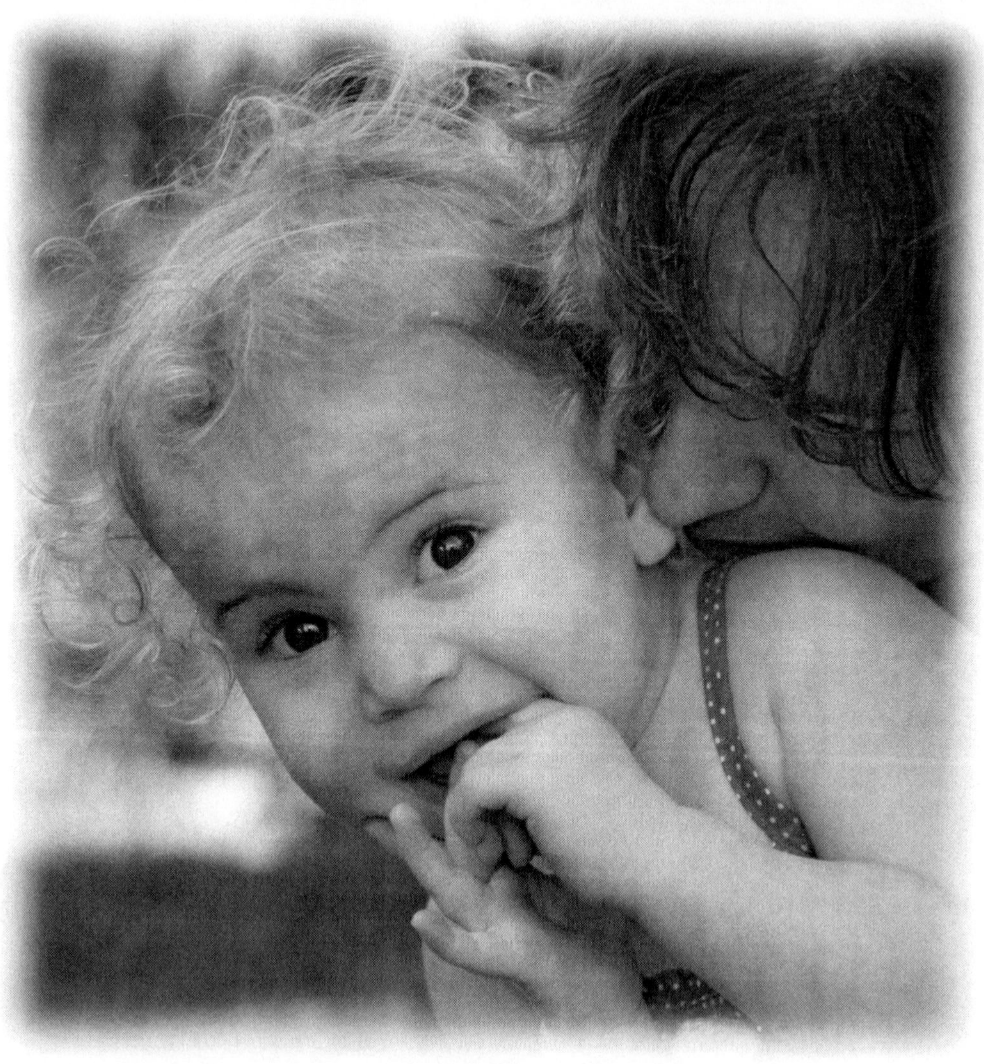

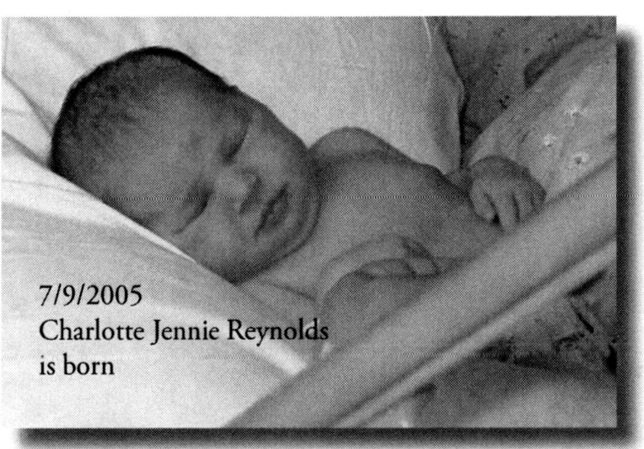

7/9/2005
Charlotte Jennie Reynolds
is born

7/12/2005
Charlotte comes home from the hospital

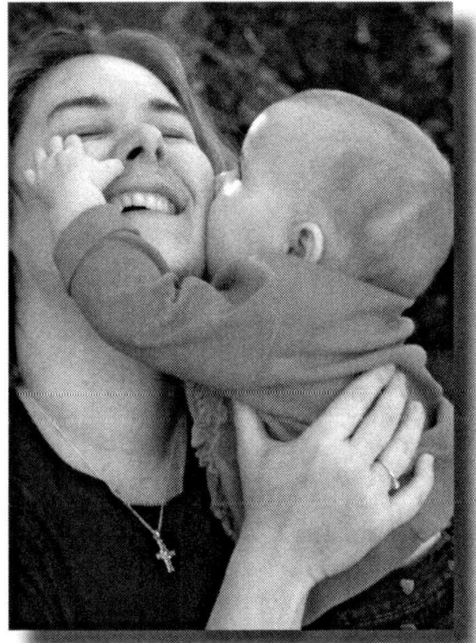

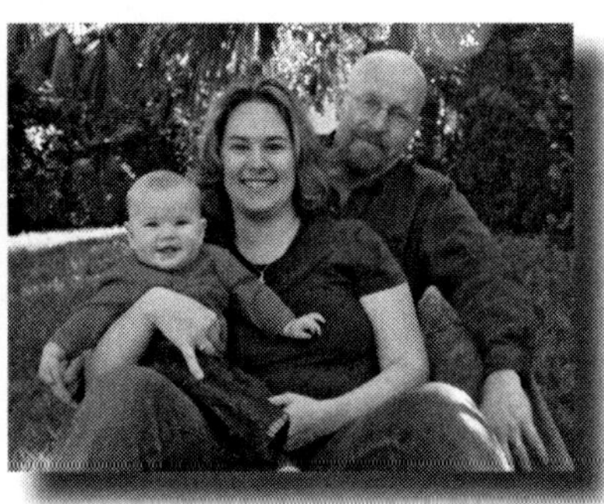

01/09/2006
Six Months Old
Photos by Jamie E. Tamm

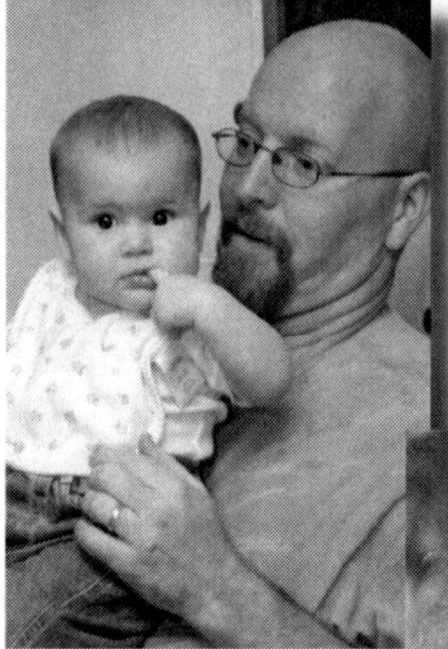

5/2006
Charlotte says her first words: mama, daddy, cat

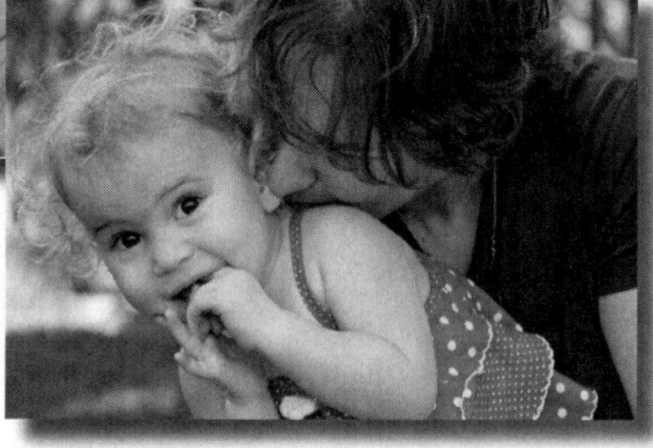

9/2006
Charlotte takes her first steps

Photos by Jamie E. Tamm

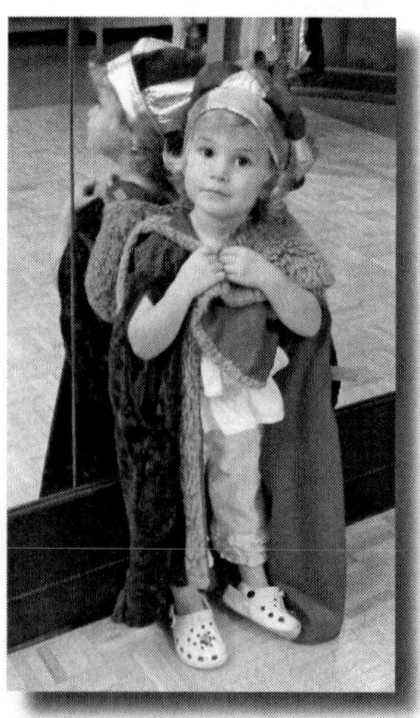

8/2007
Charlotte starts
daycare

12/1/2007
Roger and Rachel
buy Romp n' Roll

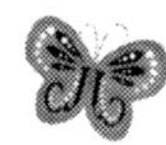

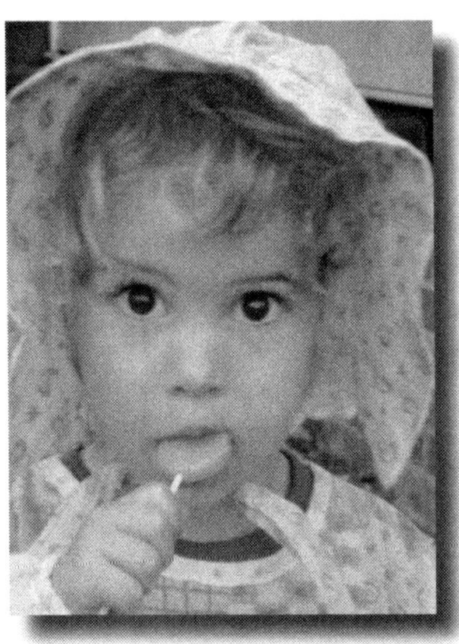

9/5/2008
Charlotte starts preschool
at Hanover Montessori

1/8/2009
Trip to Florida for Disney Marathon

1/13/2009
Return from Florida, Charlotte
starts complaining of headaches

1/20/2009
Diagnosis Day

1/21/2009
First MRI

1/22/2009
First brain surgery

1/29/2009
Second brain surgery,
insertion of Hickman

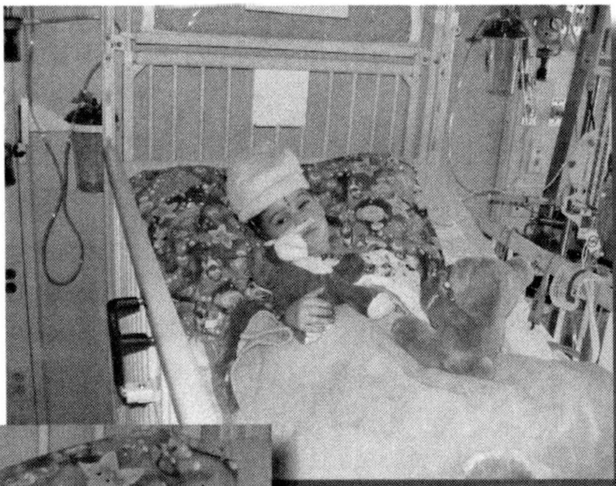

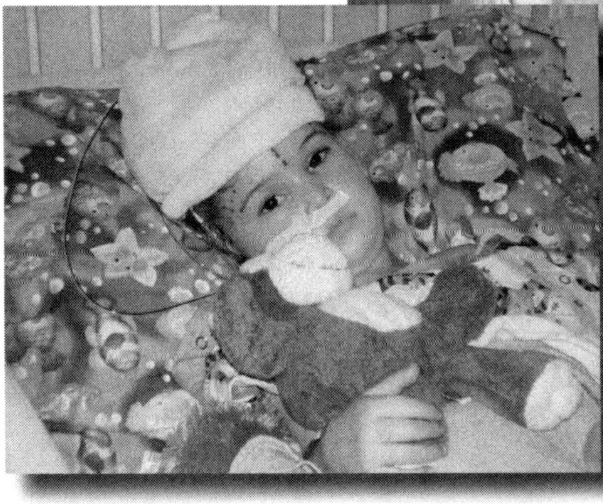

2/12/2009
Released from hospital

3/6-3/14/2009
First round of chemotherapy

3/17/2009
Admitted to hospital for abdominal
pain and neutropenic fever

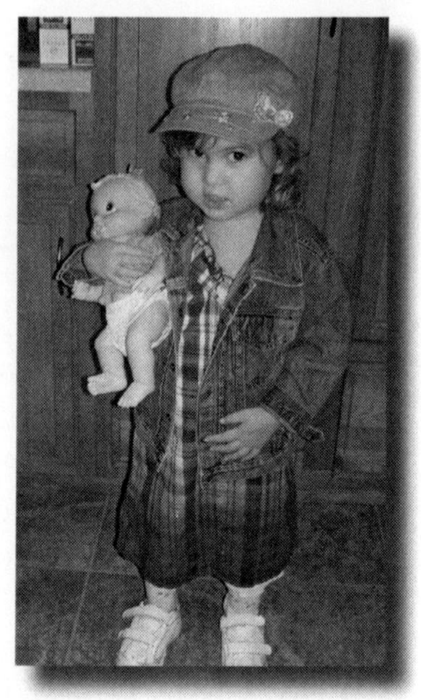

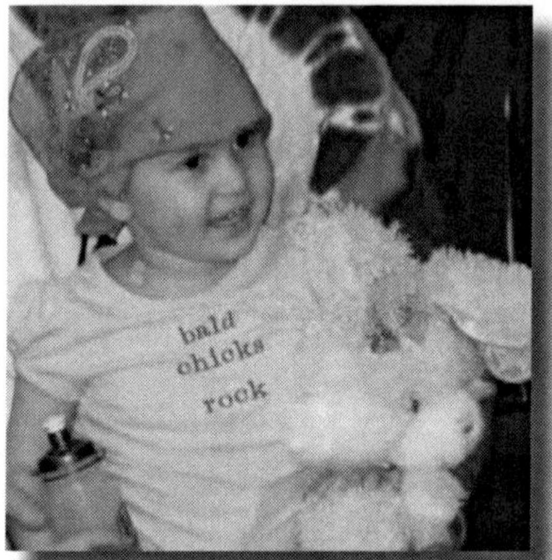

3/19/2009
Charlotte starts to lose her hair

3/23/2009
Release from hospital

4/3-4/10/2009
MRI, Second round of chemotherapy

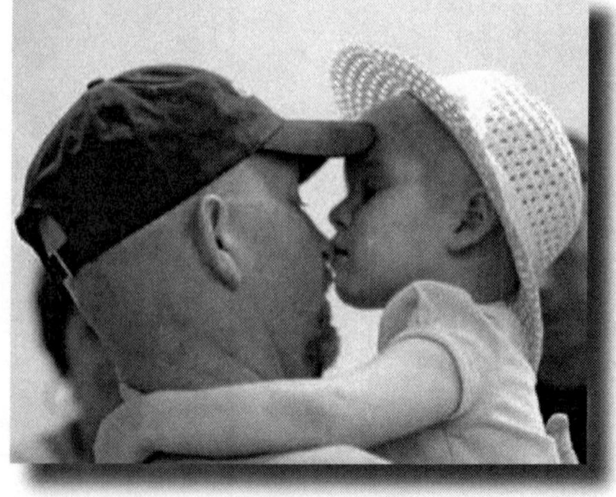

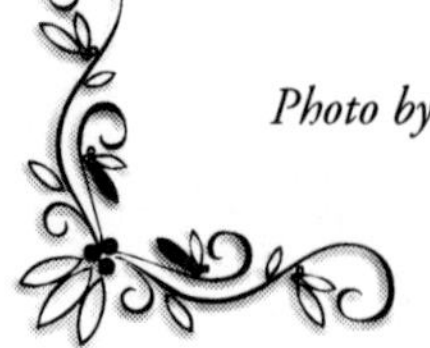

Photo by Rebecca Craig

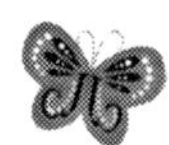

4/16-4/19/2009
Admitted for neutropenic fever

4/20 -4/24/2009
Re-admitted for infection

5/1/2009
MRI, third round of chemotherapy (stopped)

5/21/2009
Trip to Houston for 2nd opinion at MD Anderson

5/27/2009
3rd brain surgery, tumor samples sent to MD Anderson

6/18/09
Charlotte starts new protocol of chemotherapy

6/24/2009
Charlotte meets with Make-A-Wish team and sets sights on Disney

7/10/2009
Charlotte's 4th birthday party

7/11/2009
Travel to Texas

7/13/2009
Take up residence in
Ronald McDonald House in Houston, TX

7/22/2009
Proton radiation starts

Photo by Deb Harper

8/31/2009
Proton radiation ends, leave Houston and head back to VA

9/2/2009
Inconclusive MRI

9/3-11/5/2009 Outpatient chemo continues

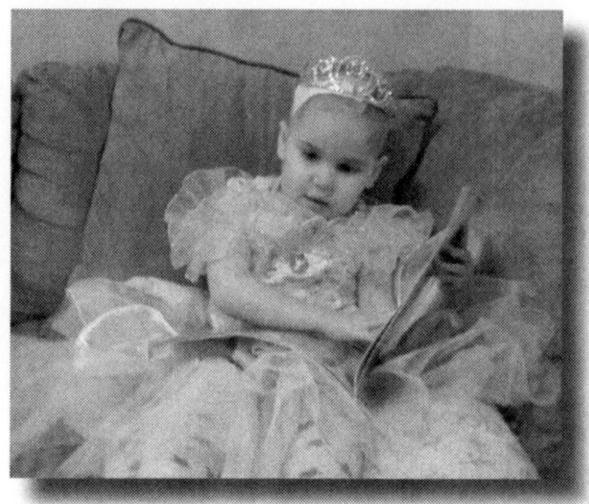

11/6/2009
Last MRI

11/7/2009
Admission to ER for
seizure

11/8/2009
Shunt surgery

11/17-11/20/09
Visits to
Smithsonian & National Zoo

11/29-11/30/2009
Trip to Baltimore Aquarium
& Steelers/Ravens game

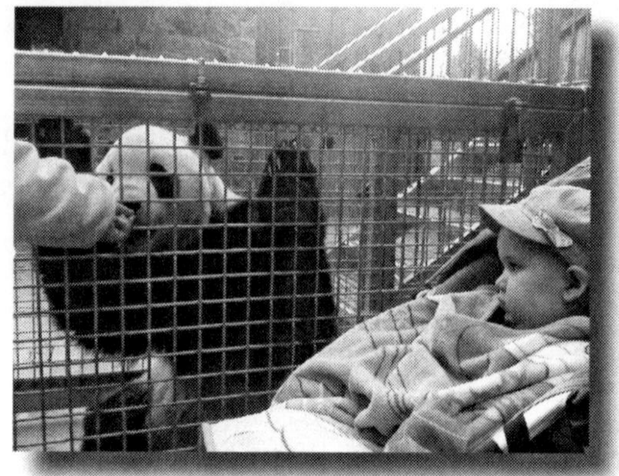

Photo by Beth Harris

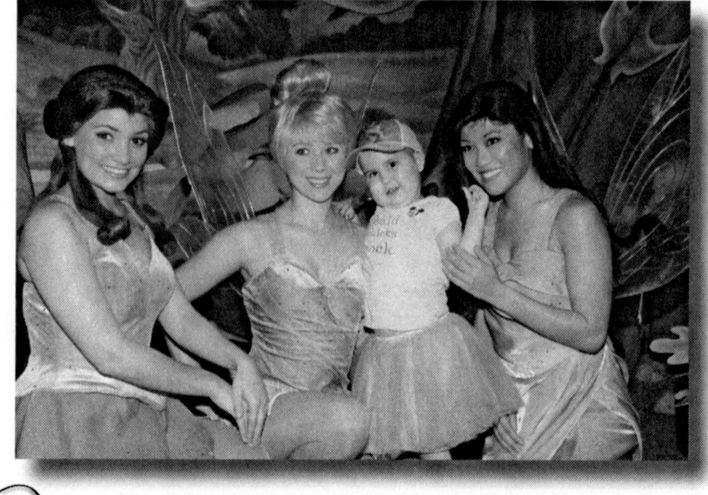

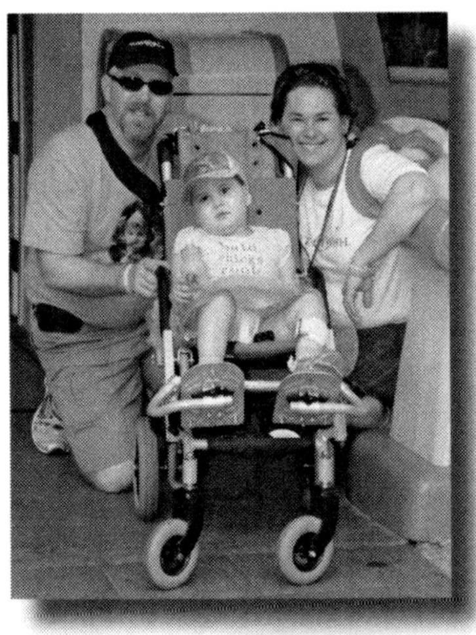

12/1-12/14/2009
Make-A-Wish trip to Florida

12/15/2009
Return to Virginia, reading vigil starts
Photos by Beth Harris

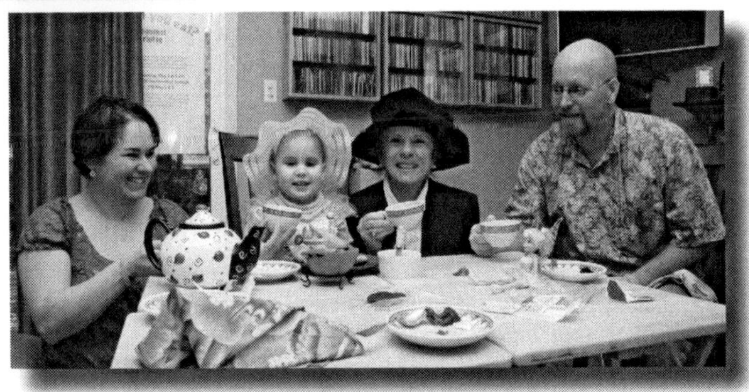

1/6/2010
CJSTUF incorporation

1/7/2010
Charlotte dies

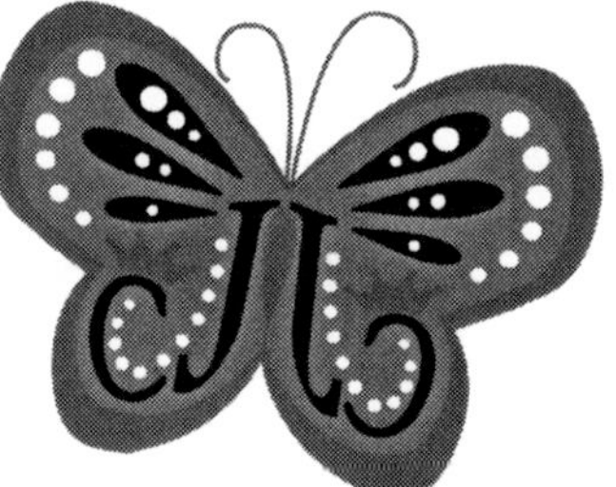

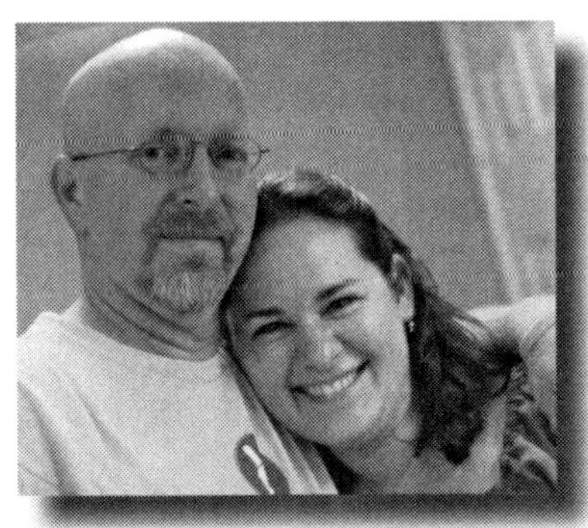

1/16/10
Charlotte's memorial service

*The "CJ Butterfly" designed
by Madison Fairburn
Photo by Britt Reints,
taken June, 2011*

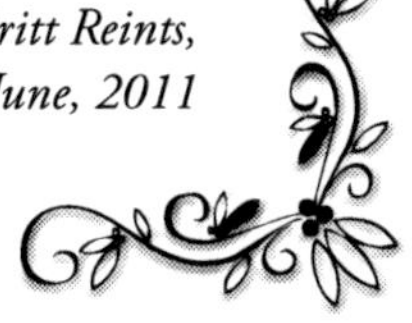

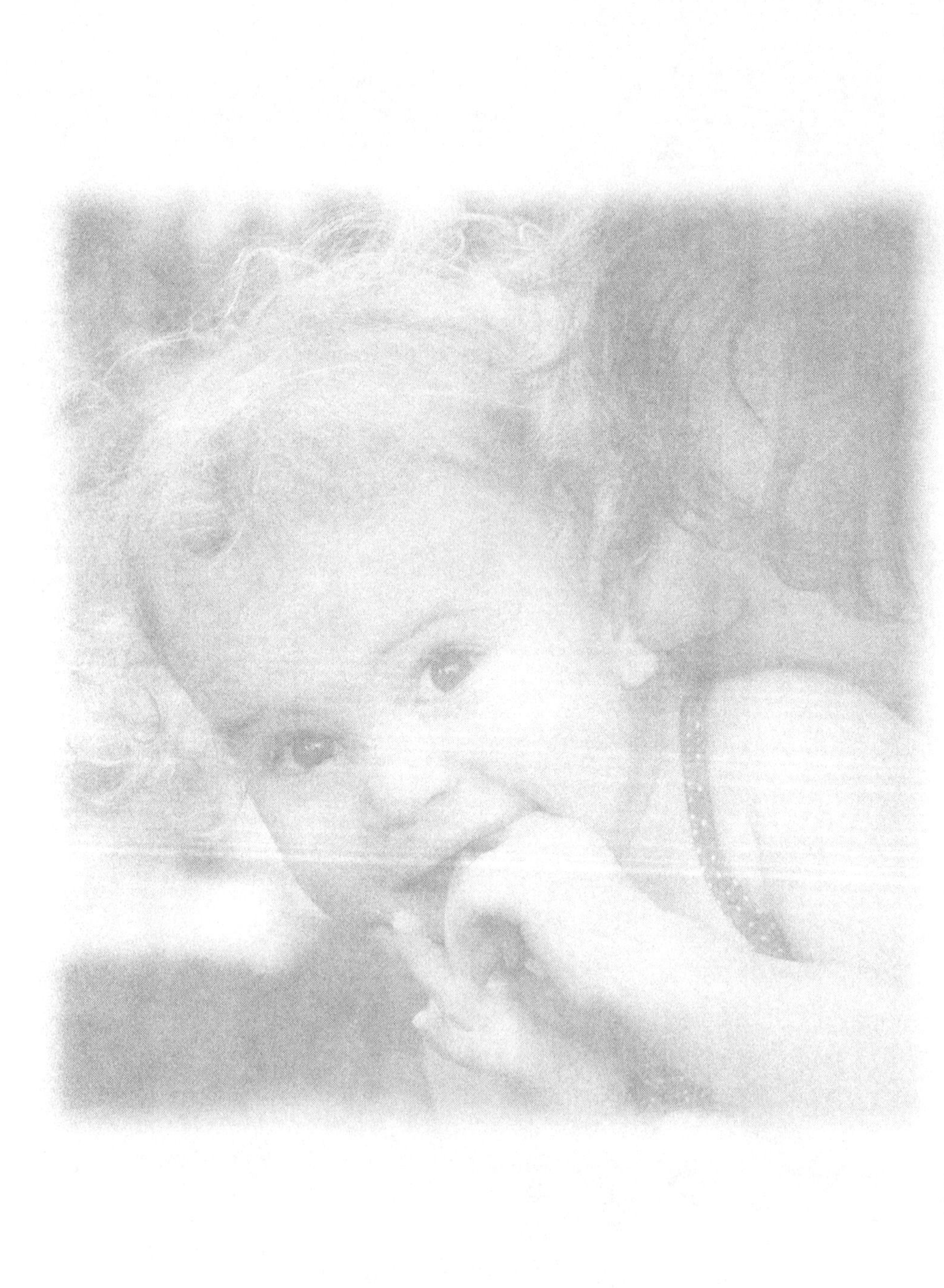

9— What Are You In For?

Once we were admitted to the hospital, we became members of an exclusive club. Unfortunately, the dues are steep and there really aren't a whole lot of perks. I'm thinking of revoking my membership but was told that all fees are non-refundable.

When you live on *Hospital Time* there is a lot of sitting and waiting. To pass the time, you often strike up conversations with complete strangers. Some of these strangers later become friends. I suppose the phrase *misery loves company* often rings true in these situations.

One of the first families that we met seemed destined to be in our circle of friends. A few days after we were admitted to the PICU, I saw this woman who looked frazzled, exhausted, and slightly familiar. We passed each other multiple times a day and I would often see her in her daughter's room. It seemed that her daughter was on a ventilator and not faring well. Many times, I started to strike up a conversation with the woman but then backed away. While Roger never shies away from conversations with strangers, I'm pretty conservative about respecting others' privacy in situations such as these. So I kept my distance.

Finally, about two weeks later, the woman approached me in the family room and said, "Do you own Romp n' Roll?"

"Um, yes, we do," I responded. "You know, I've been meaning to ask you, you look so familiar, where have I seen you before?"

The woman sighed, "We brought our son to Romp n' Roll a few weeks ago for your Open House. We signed up for the Rhythm n' Roll class on Fridays, but… well… a week later we found ourselves here. I'm Sherry. Sherry Klauer."

"Hi Sherry," I said. I introduced myself. "Is that your daughter I saw in the PICU?"

"Yes, that's Reese. She has a brain tumor. Medulloblastoma. They did a surgery to remove the tumor. It looks like they removed the tumor, but now she has posterior fossa syndrome. She's having a lot of trouble recovering. Right now she can't walk or talk."

"Oh, I'm so sorry," I responded and as our conversation progressed, we shared our similar journeys over the last few weeks. I discovered that Reese had been diagnosed only a few weeks before Charlotte. We shared the same neurosurgeon and oncology team. Before long, we knew most everything about each other's family. The Klauers had three children and six-year-old Reese was the eldest.

Over the next year, our families would follow each other through rehabilitation and cancer treatment. After Reese was released from MCV, the Klauers went to a Charlottesville hospital, one hour from their comfort zone, for intensive inpatient rehab. Reese learned to walk and talk again and Charlotte started outpatient physical and occupational therapy before beginning their respective rounds of radiation and chemotherapy. We lived only minutes from one another, saw each other frequently during clinic visits, and continued to share our joys and sorrows on each other's CaringBridge pages. Our friends joined together for a 5K Fun Run fundraiser that netted each of our families over $6000. Their son, Rhett, eventually returned to Romp n' Roll for classes. A little over a year after her diagnosis, Reese finished her treatments. Almost three years after our fateful meeting, Reese's journey to remission continues. Although her scans show no signs of tumor growth, Reese continues to require physical and occupational therapy, as well as regular visits with specialists to battle the side effects of the radiation and chemotherapy that killed her cancer cells. She is a strong survivor.

We would go on to meet other families in the hospital and in the Hematology/Oncology clinic. Each family's story was unique. Some cancer warriors were dealing with recurrences while others were close to remission. Some, like us, were newly diagnosed.

When we would see these families in the hospital or in the clinic, we would commiserate, share resources, rejoice in treatment progress, or cry with their sorrows. We met many families through CaringBridge or CarePages, a similar website. Some were local to Richmond, while others were from as far away as Wisconsin, Arizona, and Colorado.

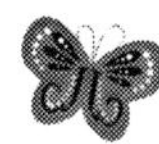

~~~~~~

Look for families who have experienced similar situations. They can provide empathy, helpful advice, and hope.

~~~~~~

We also had the opportunity to meet families who had already finished treatment. Dr. Tye introduced us to a family whose 4-year-old daughter had a tumor similar to Charlotte's and was currently in remission. We met them soon after Charlotte's first surgery and we were able to lean on them a great deal in those early months, gathering information and asking questions. Their stories allowed us to see a light at the end of a dark tunnel. They gave hope when no other hope seemed available.

We met many more families just in passing. Getting treatment in a city hospital, we saw people from all walks of life and all socioeconomic backgrounds. Many families clearly didn't have the support system or resources with which we had been blessed. It was heartbreaking to see very young children who had to be left alone in the hospital for hours on end because the parents needed to work to keep a job or insurance. There wasn't always someone who could be there with the child and the nurses couldn't keep a vigil in the room at all times. Child Life services and some volunteers certainly helped with this, but it never seemed to be enough. Thinking about this hole in the system would eventually have a deep impact on the course of our lives.

When we traveled to Houston, Texas to receive proton radiation and other services at MD Anderson Cancer Center, we met families from across the globe. As a world renowned hospital, MD Anderson had many families like ours that had reached the end of the line with their local hospital and had come to Texas seeking new or more advanced treatments. During the eight weeks that we were there, we stayed at the Ronald McDonald House, where communal living was de rigueur. This gave us ample opportunity to meet others.

As we heard another family's story, we couldn't help but empathize. Some families had been on the journey much longer than we had; others were just starting. Six months into treatment, I felt like such a veteran. Some stories were inspirational and others seemed so bleak that my heart broke. I worried if down the line my story would echo theirs. I met a 16-year-old girl who had been battling medulloblastoma with remissions and recurrences for over eight years. That was very scary.

Everyone seemed to deal with their personal trauma in their own way and we all slugged along. The parents exchanged knowing looks, sighs, and smiles. We woke up before 7:00 a.m... off to the grind of the clinic... we shuttled around to appointments all day... home to dinner. Meanwhile the kids played and laughed... and cried.

Two families in particular found their way into our inner circle. Halle was six and from Pennsylvania. Mikayla was nine and from Iowa. Like Charlotte, both girls were receiving proton radiation. Halle's appointments always followed ours, so we ended up bonding and supporting one another. Halle and Mikayla were just average kids involved in extraordinary circumstances. They both loved typical girl activities like watching *Hannah Montana*, dressing up, and shopping. They both loved crafts and music. They also both happened to have cancer.

I'm not sure why Mikayla made such an impact on Charlotte. She was the only girl and youngest child in a family of four kids. She was smart and had a quick wit. We also learned soon after meeting her that Mikayla had developed an intuitive sense of empathy far beyond her nine years. Whatever the reason, Mikayla took an immediate interest in Charlotte and, interestingly, Charlotte seemed to return the favor. About the time that we arrived at Ronald McDonald House, Charlotte was in a deeply antisocial phase. She would get inundated with attention from strangers and well-wishers and it would just get to be too much for her. For the last two months, it had been hard to watch our normally outgoing daughter retreat from social interactions, cover her face, or hide behind us when walking into a crowded room. When approached by other adults or even children, Charlotte had started to retreat inward and would sometimes just walk away.

Mikayla seemed to have the right touch, though. She never came across as loud or imposing and Charlotte seemed to appreciate that. Her approach just worked and Mikayla became the first person with whom Charlotte seemed comfortable after her social retreat. It was the first time in a long while that I saw Charlotte bond with a peer. Mikayla and Charlotte were already "bald chicks" and Halle lost her hair while we stayed in Houston. I'm not certain, but perhaps it was this inclusion in the *no hair club* that created a sense of belonging for the girls.

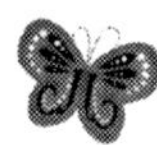

Neither Halle's mom nor I had cars in Texas. Since Mikayla's family had regular access to a large van, we frequently took all three girls on outings. It was funny to watch the heads of strangers turn as these three beautiful, bald cancer warriors went from place to place, each one a head taller than the other. The kids would talk, play, watch *Hannah Montana* movies, and make crafts. The parents would chat, cry, and complain about the latest hospital mix-up or treatment plan snafu. It was a good match.

It was during our stay in Houston that I realized that the whole childhood cancer scene can be quite the crap shoot. It seemed that for every success story with positive treatment and remission, there was at least one story of recurrence or resistance to treatment. There are leukemia patients who, by and large, follow a traditional protocol of treatment and end up with an 80% or better rate of success. Then there are the brain tumors or other cancers for which they have a moderate amount of success (60% or more), but you still hang on this precipice of recurrence with every MRI scan. You count the days until you can reach *remission* status. Even then, you don't exhale completely. Then there are cancers like Charlotte's: rare and difficult to remove. There are things that they can try. They look for solutions in every corner of the medical world, but sometimes you just run out of options. In the middle of Charlotte's treatment, we sometimes received news that another child had lost the battle. At that time, reading or hearing their stories became too painful. When we received the terminal diagnosis, though, we often found ourselves returning to these stories for solace, guidance, and even a set of benchmarks by which to gauge our own experience. Everyone's process was certainly different, but we frequently heard echoes of similar patterns in each family's story.

Although it was helpful to find others with whom we could commiserate, sometimes it was painful to witness success in other families while we continued to struggle for Charlotte's life. Sometimes we found it very difficult to be happy for the child that got an "all clear" from the doctors, rang the bell to finish treatment, had their port removed, and went home to wait for the next scan. Sometimes we found it difficult to be sympathetic to another family's challenges when our own life was such a mess. While there was a part of us that wanted to help, there was a larger part that just wanted to crawl into our hole and be left alone.

In the wake of Charlotte's passing, return visits to the hospital scene were a strange mix of comfort and anxiety. Roger seemed to find joy and purpose in visiting friends that we had met along the way when they went back into the hospital for treatments or surgeries. He still keeps up with many of the families we met during that year through their CaringBridge sites or blogs and tries to do whatever he can to *pay it forward* by bringing meals or just paying a visit. We knew how much those visits meant to us during our hospital stays and it felt good to not be on the receiving end for once. At the same time, the memories that came back every time we pulled into the hospital parking lot or checked in on the seventh-floor security gate could be painful. Charlotte was a soldier who didn't quite win the war, and it was difficult to return to the battlefield without bringing back painful memories.

10— Bringing up Baby...

"Life can only be understood looking backward.
It must be lived forward." -Soren Kierkegaard

Before Charlotte was born, well-meaning parents and friends kept repeating the same tired mantra, "You know, after your baby is born, your life is never going to be the same." Roger and I both thought this was one of the most ridiculous things anyone could say to us. Wasn't this a given? Who, in their right mind, had any idea that after a baby entered your life it would continue to be "the same"?

I distinctly remember the first few weeks of Mommyhood. I was exhausted. I was overwhelmed. Less than a week after her birth, we found ourselves back in the hospital. Charlotte had experienced latching issues with nursing and was sleeping more than she should. After three days at home, her temperature dropped to dangerous levels and we faced our first visit to the emergency room. The official diagnosis was *failure to thrive*. After multiple tests, including a spinal tap that forced my post-partum hormones off the deep end, the doctors couldn't seem to come up with a definitive diagnosis but recommended a course of IV antibiotics. Whatever the cause, this seemed to do the trick. Within 24 hours, Charlotte's eating improved. Gradually, the nursing got easier. After a few more days, we returned home.

Early in the journey with cancer, we found many comparisons between the whole experience and having a newborn baby: the sleepless nights, the anxiety of the unknown, the hospital experience, everyone rallying around and wanting to help. It's just a little more extreme and intense. OK, it's *a lot* more extreme and intense, and there are fewer people who have actually been through it.

When you are a first-time parent, information, advice, offers to help, and important decisions that must be made can be overwhelming. Do you feed the child by breast or bottle? Does she sleep in the crib or do we co-sleep? Comfort or cry it out? When do you begin solids? How often do you change her diaper? Is she teething or is she getting sick? Or is she just unhappy? For every question, you can find a wide range of opinions. If you look to the parenting section at your local bookstore, you will find shelves of books on a multitude of topics and each book seems to contradict the next. With all these options, what is a new parent to do?

In our early parenting experiences, Roger and I sought balance above all else. We learned from our own parents, other family members, and our close friends. We watched the parenting styles of others and we decided what we liked and what we didn't like. We learned what seemed to work for us. It was all about balance. Our approach to these early experiences was with flexibility and Charlotte's best interest in mind. We kept that philosophy going throughout her struggle with cancer as well.

The first time we both left Charlotte at the hospital for a few hours, it was like leaving her as an infant all over again. Either Roger or I had been by Charlotte's side almost constantly since her diagnosis and we definitely needed a break. We scheduled a much-needed date to celebrate Roger's birthday. Charlotte was still in the Pediatric ICU and it had only been about three days since her second brain surgery. We knew we would not be gone for a long time, but we still fretted over every little detail. We left notes about what to do in any situation, paying extra close attention to our cell phones should anyone call, and spent the whole date pretty much talking about her. We didn't seem to think about the fact that she was in a Pediatric ICU, under the supervision of doctors and nurses who actually could do a better job caring for her at this point than we could. As time went on and we needed to leave Charlotte with various sitters (whether it was family or friends), we found the process did get easier.

Probably the most significant effect of Charlotte's brain surgeries was the motor weakness that developed on her left side. Based on the neurosurgeon's expertise and the path he had to use to de-bulk the tumor, we were warned that the left side of her body could be significantly weakened, if not paralyzed, following the surgery. We anticipated the results of the first surgery, hoping for the best but preparing ourselves for the worst.

When she emerged from the first surgery, Charlotte was certainly weak, but we were thrilled that she was able to move her left side with some encouragement. She even crossed her legs for the doctor on command. She

had some facial asymmetry and struggled to support herself in an upright position. The left side of her face drooped slightly so that her adorable smile was just a little crooked. She also could not grip or release with her left hand. Fortunately, Charlotte had always favored her right hand for eating and writing, but this weakness made tasks that required the use of two hands (fine motor control and bilateral coordination) very difficult. After about two weeks, Charlotte was starting to sit up with support and started to walk *very* small distances with significant assistance. Weeks and months of physical therapy and occupational therapy followed, targeting the motor skills on her left side.

It was odd to have to do a lot of things for Charlotte that she had become so proficient in before her diagnosis. We had to help her eat again and had to help her get dressed. She needed a booster seat and a bedrail for safety, items that we had long ago abandoned and passed along to others. She needed help navigating stairs and we had to use a stroller for even the shortest distances.

One of the most disappointing and frustrating parts of this process was Charlotte's regression with potty training. We had worked so fastidiously and halfway through her third year Charlotte was finally pretty much potty trained, except at night. She was wearing "big girl underwear" every day, with very few accidents. All of this ended after our first night in the hospital. Between all the fluids being pumped into her tiny body, having her hooked up to multiple IVs, wires, and other telemetry, and the subsequent surgeries that left her immobile for days at a time, it was just not possible for her to use the bathroom normally. As the weeks passed and we prepared for procedures like necessary catheterizations, the inpatient chemotherapy that required 100 cc of fluid to pump through her system every hour, and even *more* invasive procedures, we eventually resigned ourselves to going back to diapers.

Somewhere along the way, as Charlotte started gaining more independence, we thought we might introduce the concept of potty training again. Boy, were we wrong. This was one of the few elements of her life in which she had control and she was *not* going to relinquish that control to anyone. We tried bribes, enticements, motivation, and even peer pressure. Certainly by this point, all of her peers were potty trained. We even tried telling her that she couldn't go to Disney World until she was wearing underwear because Disney World didn't allow diapers. She didn't bat an eye at this thinly-veiled threat.

One day, my mother was discussing this concept with her and said, "You know, Charlotte, all your friends use the big girl potty and wear underwear."

Charlotte looked up, rolled her eyes, and said in a voice more reflective of a 14-year-old, "SO?" At that point, I think I just gave up. She would use the potty when she was ready, not a day sooner. And if this was the one thing that gave her some control, I would keep changing her diapers until *she* was ready. Maybe on some level, Charlotte knew something that we didn't know: she didn't need to be potty trained. Her life was so short that there were many other things that she needed to accomplish. She didn't need to put *potty trained* on her resume.

While regularity had never been an issue in her life before, Charlotte struggled with constipation almost constantly after her cancer diagnosis. Frequent anesthesia, certain medications, and many of the chemotherapy agents cited constipation as a main side effect. Couple this with her inability to move a great deal and her limited appetite or diet, and Charlotte was far from "regular." Early on, the medical team tried many different strategies to induce a bowel movement including laxatives, stool softeners, fluids, flax meal, fruits and juices, and high-fiber supplements. As we posted our struggles in our online blog, friends, family, and strangers would offer up their tips and tricks for poop induction. Alas, at one point during our first hospitalization, it became necessary to administer the first of more than a few enemas. This was certainly a last resort but a necessary one as her belly was extremely distended and she was in obvious discomfort. We had already tried everything else.

As we sat by Charlotte's bedside waiting for the enema to work on her tiny body, Roger and I were instantly transported back to our childbirth experience. I have never had an enema but seeing her in pain and, more importantly, seeing Roger's response to her pain, I was suddenly back in the delivery room 3 ½ years ago. The heart racing, the cramping, the crying, and through it all, Roger was calm, quiet, and an oasis of peace. He held her hand, rubbed her forehead, distracted her by singing her favorite songs, and reminded her to *breathe...* modeling all the while. Roger was a fabulous labor coach when I gave birth and that calming demeanor just continued to shine through as a beacon of comfort for Charlotte.

Later, as Charlotte's time on earth waned, she began to sleep more and more. In her final days, her sleeping time increased and the time that she was awake and alert became shorter and shorter. She gradually lost her ability to walk, her ability to talk, and her ability to eat; however, she never seemed to lose her awareness of the world around her. Even in those quiet moments

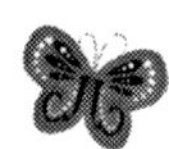

when we thought she was a breath away from death, she would react with the slightest finger squeeze, eye flutter, or twitch as we talked, sang, and read to her.

In those moments, I was again brought back to the intensity of the birth experience. We kept vigil by her side, knowing that at any point things could change. We knew what the typical progression of the disease would look like, but nobody had an exact timetable. It was like waiting to go into labor. As the process went on, we grew tired, cranky, and impatient, but we didn't want to leave because at any moment, *it could happen*. Like childbirth, we knew, scientifically, what to expect. We also knew that nature had a way of taking its own course and we had to trust the process as it happened. We couldn't rush the experience any more than we could slow it down.

As Charlotte drifted towards death, she also drifted back towards infancy. As parents, we never wanted to miss a moment. We were exhausted by the process, but we hung on every possible opportunity to be there with her.

People keep asking us if we'll ever have another baby. It seems we already have. We've had the same one twice.

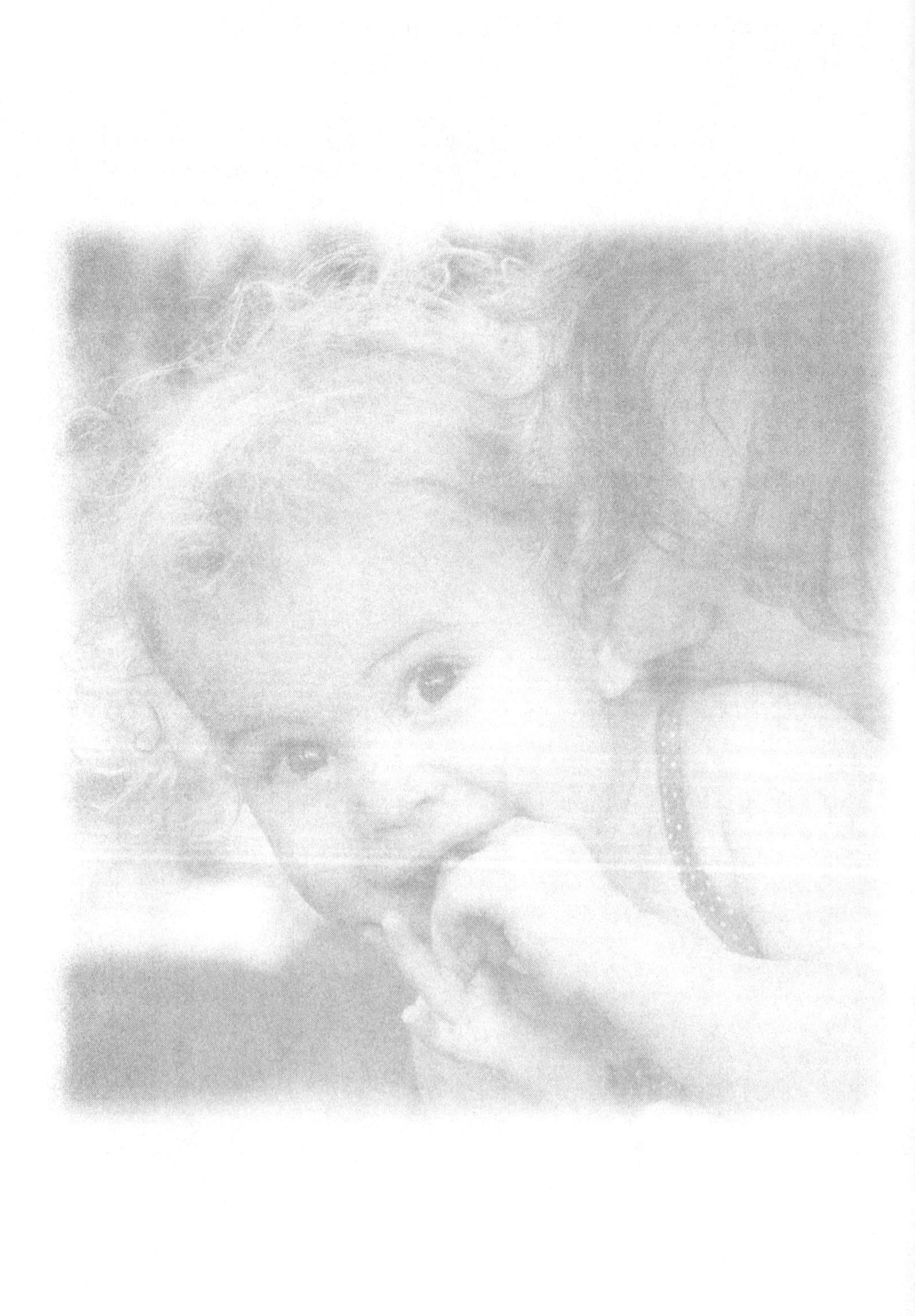

11— On the Other Side of the Table

"It's hard enough to work and raise a family when your kids are all healthy and relatively normal, but when you add on some kind of disability or disease, it can just be such a burden."
—*Actress Patricia Heaton*

Charlotte loved to be outside. Maybe it's because she was born in July. From an early age, we took her for walks in the stroller or swaddled in the sling or Baby Bjorn. When she first started toddling around, she practiced taking those first hesitant steps in the soft grass of our front yard. Although she was crawling by nine months, it took another six months before she decided to let go of a grown-up hand or a push toy and walk on her own. She adopted this "monkey walk" where she would walk on her hands with her bottom pointed to the sky. She could get anywhere she needed with the monkey walk so what was her motivation to walk upright like the rest of us?

One day in late September, at about fifteen months of age, Charlotte decided she was ready. With camcorder in hand, we captured her first hesitant steps on her own as she let go of the car she was pushing and toddled around our cul-de-sac. Once she had mastered this task, it wasn't long before she was climbing and running on everything.

We had a park around the corner from our house and Charlotte visited the park almost every day that the weather allowed. She was never scared of the big ladders or the slippery slides. We usually had to watch carefully because she would get herself stuck somewhere at the top of the jungle gym and not know how to navigate her way down.

Daily recreation at Romp n' Roll only served to further her physical development. By the time she was a little over two years old, Charlotte could scale a small rock wall, swing on a trapeze and navigate an obstacle course like nobody's business. It seemed that Charlotte had avoided inheriting my klutz gene. Her physical development was moving along just fine.

Three months after Charlotte's first brain surgery, we were still working to recover from the motor weaknesses that resulted from the invasive medical procedure. She walked with a brace but still struggled to climb stairs, coordinate her movements, or sustain energy for long periods of time. At a benefit dinner in April, we realized the true extent of her physical limitations. Some of the kids, including Charlotte, went to play on the playground. We saw children younger and smaller than her running around on the equipment and moving up and down the ladders or poles without hesitation; Charlotte, on the other hand, had to move more cautiously. The best example was the slide. The steps were easy for her to manage and designed in such a way to be very easily navigated by everyone, but the slides themselves were a different story. They had a handle at the top so children could grab it, swing under, and drop down the slide really fast. I saw several kids do this, including kids who hadn't quite turned two. On the other hand, as Charlotte got up to the top, it was a challenge just to sit down and push her body over the edge.

We had gotten so used to the way she was and had been so impressed by how far she had come since the surgery that we lost sight of how far we still had to go before she could keep up with her peers. What's odd is that it didn't make me sad or feel sorry for myself or anyone else. It was just another one of those reality checks. It also showed us that the therapies in which we had enrolled Charlotte were still necessary if she was going to keep up with the other kids.

Sometimes when we saw that Charlotte understood her physical limitations and how they differentiated her from her friends, it didn't seem to bother her. There were other times on playgrounds, at Romp n' Roll, or during other playdates where she tried to keep up and grew frustrated by the differences. She tried to climb stairs, walk fast, jump, and use her balance but was hampered by her inability to do the things that her friends could do.

Her therapy regimen was very scattered during those first few months. Inpatient chemotherapy, frequent unexpected hospitalizations, and our trip to Houston for radiation all delayed regular therapy opportunities. Once we returned to Virginia in September of 2009, it was time to renew our efforts with therapy full force. After only about two weeks of regular therapy, we already started to see improvement in her grasp, release, and walking abilities. It was around this time that the insurance coverage for her therapy ran out. We had exhausted the cap for what insurance would cover and had begun to pay for therapy out of pocket. At the same time, we initiated the process by

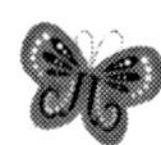

which Charlotte would be able to receive similar services through our county school system.

As a speech language pathologist, my career had been devoted to working with individuals with special needs. I knew the law and understood the system inside and out. This provided a huge advantage to us as we navigated this process. In the first place, I knew that since Charlotte's motor weaknesses would have a profound impact on her ability to participate in general education activities with other children, she should qualify for special education services, including her requisite therapies. I also knew who to call and how to go about receiving an evaluation that would lead to eligibility for services. At the same time, it was still somewhat bizarre to sit on the other side of the table, listening to professionals evaluate my daughter, discuss her strengths and weaknesses, and make recommendations for future treatment.

Many people are familiar with the five stages of grief, popularized and eloquently explained by Elisabeth Kübler-Ross in her 1969 book *On Death and Dying*. If you missed that psychology lesson, the stages are: *Denial, Anger, Bargaining, Depression,* and *Acceptance*. If you have experienced the loss of a close friend, family member, or even a family pet, you have probably gone through these grief stages. There is no set time in which you should or should not stay in each of the stages. There is no set order, either. The principle of the stages of grief is that before you reach true *Acceptance*, you must traverse at some point all the other stages. For some, it is a quick trip and for others it is a long journey. Some get stuck in *Depression, Anger, or Denial,* and truly, some may never even reach *Acceptance*.

What you may not realize is that you don't have to experience physical death to endure the five stages of grief. Grief can be borne out of any kind of loss. Realizing that your child is not *perfect* in some way, shape, or form is a loss. I am not talking about those cute little imperfections or personality traits that make your kid a unique individual. I am talking about disability or disease.

I have seen this intimately with parents who have a child with autism. When a child is diagnosed with a developmental disability, there is a sense of loss. The child is no longer 'typical.' It does not mean that they will not experience success and it does not mean that they will not have a full and happy life. It doesn't mean that the parents love this child any less, but it does mean that the family will never, ever experience the prototypical lifestyle of the average family. That life, as they might have known it, is over. Instead, the family must work to overcome the loss the best way they know how. This often takes the form of treatments, therapy, intensive counseling, medication, hospitalizations… the list could go on. Along the journey, the family will experience their own set of grief stages. Some get stuck in *Denial* and end up with unreasonable expectations for their child with serious challenges. Some fixate on *Anger* and it comes through with contentious meetings with members of the special education team. Some end up with *Depression* and this often leads to divorce, frustration, or other personal challenges. Others work through these stages and come out on the other side. Their world is not sunshine and roses all the time; these families still experience significant challenges every day. But they have accepted their child for who he or she is, and they have accepted their life as it is. They work each day to make it better and take each educational plan, each behavior plan, each therapy session, and each school year one day at a time.

> **If your child does require extensive assistance due to a medical illness or injury, he or she may also qualify for special education services in the public schools. Contact your local school district to find out more.**

I now feel a new kinship for these families. Although I always felt that I could empathize and relate to their experiences, I now *know* their struggles from the inside out. We were not just grieving the fact that Charlotte had a life-threatening condition. We were grieving the loss of what once was. We were grieving the fact that she struggled with things that were once easy for her. We were grieving the struggles that we endured in our attempt to achieve whatever sense of normalcy we could find.

I think Roger summarized these feelings well when he created this post on CaringBridge only a few weeks after her diagnosis:

On January 20, 2009, a 50-ton boulder came crashing into our house. There was a lot of damage, some injuries, and much chaos and confusion but after the dust clears, someone will come in, clear away the rock and debris, and rebuild the house. It will probably be a very different house and we'll always know where the patches are but we'll get through it.

Someone in a more chronic situation, such as a child with autism or a serious birth defect also has that 50-ton boulder in their house but this one is very slowly moving around the house, constantly, and endlessly crushing everything. You can get out of the way of the worst of it but you'll never save the coffee table or that lamp Aunt Edna gave you and man, does it do a number on the toes.

Then there are those who have no house for their boulder to crush. The list can go on and on. This situation could be much worse and no matter what happens, we'll make the best of it.

Charlotte's (and our) experience with the special education process never made it past the evaluation stage. Before we could get to eligibility, her diagnosis was deemed terminal. I will never forget, however, how it felt to sit on the other side of the table, advocating for my child with special needs and feeling so grateful that these services existed.

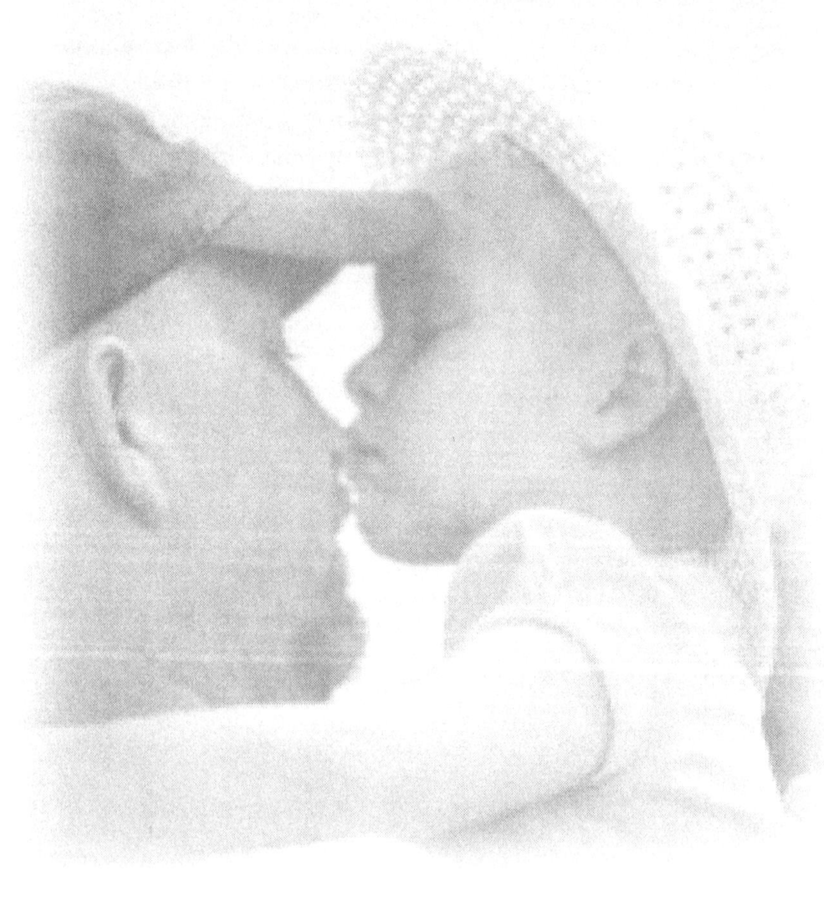

Lesson #4: Think twice before you speak.

One evening, fairly early into our year with cancer, I came into Romp n' Roll from the pharmacy frustrated because some of Charlotte's prescriptions did not get filled correctly. I was obviously agitated and a parent who knew of our situation asked what was wrong. I tried to tell her and basically ended by saying I was having a really rough day. She replied, "Well, it could be worse." Really? You're going to tell the parent of a kid with a brain tumor who just finished major surgery and is getting ready for rounds of chemotherapy that "it could be worse"? Worse than what? How could it really be worse? And do I even want to think about what that would look like?

The corollary to this rule is the use of the phrase "At least." You encounter this in different ways, but it is most often associated with the grief phase, i.e. once a child's condition is deemed terminal or when they die. I don't think I personally experienced this to a great extent, but I know other parents have. Think about some of these dreaded phrases:

- *At least* you still have other children

- *At least* you can still have children

- *At least* you now know that she is in a better place

- *At least* it was caught early. Kids are really resilient, you know. She will bounce back.

When you are the parent of a terminally ill or deceased child, there is no *at least.* This is not the time to count blessings. Sometimes it is just important to be allowed to grieve the loss for what it is. These well-intentioned words do not comfort or heal.

There are other phrases that can make families dealing with chronic or terminal illness twinge. Things like "God doesn't give anyone more than they can bear", "God must have needed another angel", or "He's in a better place now" might seem comforting in your head but often those words are like fingernails on a chalkboard to the grieving family.

It is also interesting how people will ask very personal questions or offer unsolicited advice. Their intention may be to help, but they usually only evoke frustration or anger from the intended recipient. I have heard things like, "So, how's your marriage?" or "You need to be strong for (family member)" or "At least you're young and can have more children."

If you've been in this situation, you could probably cite a laundry list of similar quotes. Interestingly, what bothers one person may not really be annoying or offensive to another since everyone is in a different place with their grief process. We commiserated with other families who heard even more ridiculous things.

As logic might dictate, the most empathic people were those who had been in similar situations. While very few people had actually walked in *our* shoes, we encountered many who had faced some type of journey in the cancer world. Either they were cancer survivors or they had a loved one who had fought (and sometimes lost) the battle. I would say that, for the most part, their ability to empathize was true to form. We did encounter a few individuals who didn't seem to experience life with cancer the same way and seemed hell-bent on making sure you knew it.

I had one acquaintance from college, we will call her Amanda, who reconnected with me during this time. She proceeded to send me emails documenting her mother's very sad and very painful journey with brain cancer. Amanda's emails were definitely unsolicited and consisted largely of graphic, painful descriptions of her mother's death and all of the sadness and pain that she experienced in the process of her mother's death and burial. I think that Amanda's intention was to show that she could empathize with my situation and that she could be a person to lean on if I felt the need to talk with someone. In reality, it only served to sadden me further and did not ease my pain in any way.

12— It Can Always Get Worse

"When you're going through Hell, keep going."
—Winston Churchill

So you've gotten a pretty good picture of our life in 2009 so far. We spent our time in and out of hospitals. We lived each day dealing with the anxiety of the unknown related to our child's mortality. In between all of that we tried to balance other aspects of our domestic and professional lives. Did you catch the part where I said never tell a parent of a child with cancer, "It could be worse"?

Can you believe that it got worse?

On top of everything medical that we needed to deal with, we were running a business during one of the worst recessions in American history. Although the business had seen great success before we purchased it, apparently we bought just as the economy tanked. We kept many of our loyal customers; however, others had to move away or stop coming to classes due to layoffs and job transfers. Kids' classes and parties became an expendable indulgence rather than a necessity to some and our revenue dropped by almost 20 percent. I still felt relatively lucky because we lived in a state that didn't have nearly the foreclosures, unemployment rates, or other financial woes that other regions of the country seemed to be experiencing, but the cumulative effect of the national news and both real and imagined financial anxiety in our region made it even more difficult to market our business. At a time when we should have been devoting even more hands-on time to our jobs, we had to cut back to care for Charlotte's needs.

Before her diagnosis, both Roger and I had taken a few freelance jobs on the side to help make ends meet. It was rough and we were both working upwards of 60 hours a week, but we were squeaking by. By the end of January, we had to give up almost all of these additional sources of income aside from Roger's occasional music gigs.

While we managed to pay our household bills with our marginal income and support from family and friends, the business continued to operate at a loss and we maxed out our credit cards trying to keep the business afloat.

But wait. There's more.

We had other family members facing health issues. My mom went to the hospital twice during visits to Virginia due to recurrent, debilitating asthma attacks. Both times, the ambulance had to be called to the house and one time they had to rule out a heart attack with a heart catheterization. In September we learned that my stepfather needed to have a heart valve replaced. Originally we thought the surgery could be delayed for a few years, but he ended up having open heart surgery the day we left for Florida for our Make-A-Wish trip in December. He was on the mend during our visit.

Sometime in November, I opened the front door of our house, getting ready for a visit from a friend, and found Punkin, one of our three cats, dead on the front porch! Apparently he had been there for a few days. We rarely used our front door and, with everything else going on, we hadn't really noticed that he was missing. The cats hung around outside mostly and since all three cats were orange tabbies, it was easy to not notice that one was missing. Tigger, one of the other cats, had apparently been trying to tell us all week. I had wondered why his loud meowing had become exceedingly annoying in recent days. All of a sudden it was clear. When I found Punkin, I screeched and Roger quickly took care of the situation. He placed Punkin in an old pillowcase and buried him in the backyard. It seemed that while he wasn't very old, his heart just must have given out because he didn't seem to have suffered any trauma. Charlotte used to say, "I have three cats: Tigger, Punkin, and Noah. Noah comes inside, but Tigger and Punkin' stay outside." Well, from that point on, Punkin was *permanently* outside.

Then there were the very fun dealings with the insurance company. Has anyone experienced significant hospitalization and not had *some* kind of difficulty with the insurance company? Because we were self-employed, we had our own private insurance. For that I was very grateful since we didn't have to make the decision, as many parents do, to keep hours at their job just so they could keep insurance coverage. Our policy was a high-deductible policy, so once we paid our $5000 deductible almost everything was covered. Charlotte racked up over $800,000 in medical expenses that year between hospitalizations, chemotherapy, radiation, other medications, and surgeries. I think we paid for less than 10% of that out of our own pocket and much of our out-of-pocket expenses were covered through money that we received via the fundraisers and other individual donations. While I was grateful that we had insurance, the bureaucracy was difficult to manage during our family crisis.

My chief issue was that we just had to double and triple check everything. There was a great deal of confusion at the beginning as to whether our primary hospital was in-network or out-of-network. This made a huge difference in our out-of-pocket cost and we kept getting different answers from our hospital and the insurance company. It took multiple phone calls, documentation, and often re-filing of a few claims to make sure that the insurance company paid everything that they were supposed to pay.

Keep insurance papers and receipts in a three-ring binder or expandable file for easy reference.

When we went to MD Anderson, there was more confusion about our in-network/out-of-network status. Apparently the hospital was in-network but some of the doctors we saw were not. We worked with some fabulous employees in the billing department who helped us navigate the paperwork and appeals. Without them, our out-of-pocket expenses would have been considerably higher.

At one point Charlotte's protocol called for three rounds of stem cell transplants with high-dose chemotherapy. These procedures typically involve a two-to-three-week hospital stay that includes rounds of chemotherapy in higher than usual concentrations followed by stem cell transplants (the patient's own cells that had been harvested previously) to replace the destroyed bone marrow. Each round is spaced about a month apart and neutropenic fevers and intermediate hospitalizations between rounds are typical.

So here was the situation: although our local hospital was finally confirmed to be in-network for all of Charlotte's usual medical care, it was not an in-network hospital for *transplants*. The closest hospital considered in-network was Duke in North Carolina, which was over three hours away. The insurance company gave us two options. We could relocate to Duke for essentially at least three months. It would be difficult to determine whether

Charlotte could even go back and forth between Duke and home during treatments so we would probably end up there for a while. Of course, this would really mean that Charlotte and *one of her parents* would go since the other one had to stay and care for the business. Who wanted to make that choice?

The other option would be to stay at our primary hospital, 30 minutes from our home. She could receive all of the same care from the same team of doctors. We would have access to everyone in *The Network* for emotional and tangible support as well as our counselors, social workers, doctors, nurses, and other professionals that had become our team, but we would have to pay the out-of-network cost which could run up to $40,000 per round.

Which option would you choose?

As I related this story to *The Network*, I was greeted with disbelief and anger. It seemed utterly ridiculous to everyone… except the insurance company. I sought help from our state insurance commission. The ombudsman was wonderful. He heard my story, felt we had a case, and made some phone calls. With his help, we filed two appeals that included letters from both Dr. Khan and Dr. Tye explaining why staying in Virginia was a better solution. Our hospital even agreed to match any costs that Duke would charge making the net cost to the insurance company a wash. The insurance company would have actually come out ahead because going to Duke would involve reimbursement of travel expenses.

Strangely, despite two appeals and all the logic this side of a mathematician's doctoral thesis, the insurance company maintained its stance. To their credit, everyone I ever talked to at the insurance company was polite, sympathetic, and responsive. We just didn't get the response that we desired. We received the second denial letter about the same time that we also received news that the current chemotherapy protocol wasn't working. All of our appeals and frustration seemed to be for naught as we now had to look in a completely different direction for treatment options.

Interestingly, this situation was what motivated *The Network* into a fundraising frenzy. The funds that were raised were still needed for travel expenses and incidental medical bills so nothing was wasted; however, it was that initial ire at the insurance company's stringent adherence to *policy* that ignited the fervent desire in our friends and family to offer assistance.

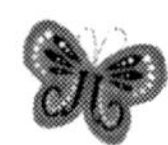

In the end, many of these little bumps in the road in and of themselves were not monumental; however, given our situation, the effects were magnified. When you're driving down the road in a 2009 Cadillac Escalade (Hybrid, of course), it's smooth sailing; even if you hit a pothole, you can keep cruising along. But we were riding in a beat-up 1978 Chevy Nova with a rebuilt transmission, we had logged over 200,000 miles, and we were barely passing inspection. We felt *every* little bump in the road and we were on a cross-country trip with very few exit ramps. Even the littlest thing could be upsetting.

As the year went on, the bad news just seemed to pile up. We didn't get nearly enough good news to counteract the frustration we felt every time something didn't go according to plan. All of this drama seemed to reach a peak as we approached the end of summer and journeyed into fall.

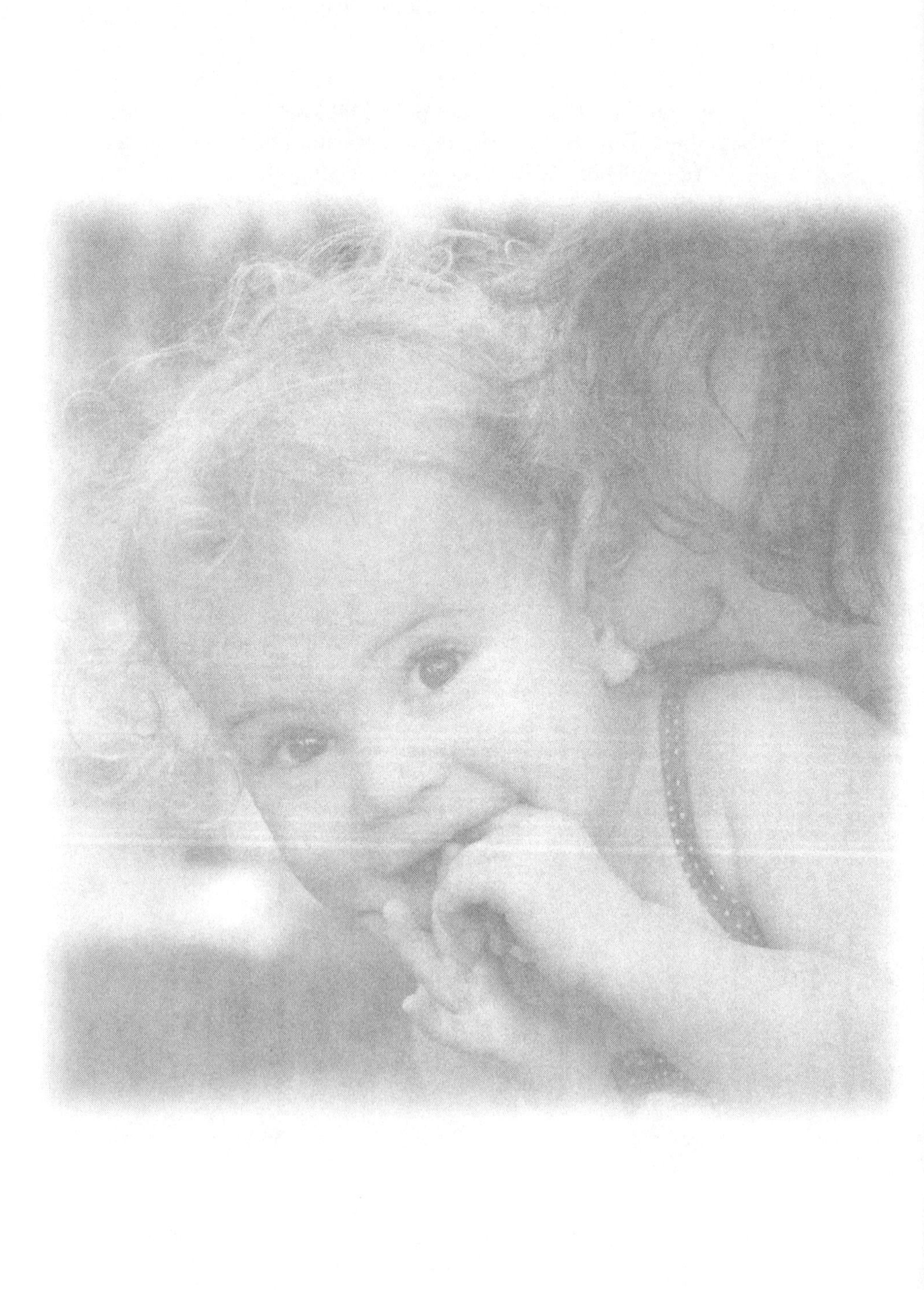

13— The Journey to the Terminal

"I'm dying. So are you. The process is just accelerated in me."
--Author Christopher Hitchens on his battle with esophageal cancer

At the end of the summer, we returned from Texas to reassess the plan. Unfortunately, we were still filled with anxiety. There was a lot to consider as we anticipated the results of all the medical intervention Charlotte had experienced over the last eight weeks. We came home looking for answers, but we seemed to face more questions.

Excerpts from one of Roger's CaringBridge entries might help to set the scene:

9/8/2009

On Thursday, July 30, 2009, Chicago White Sox pitcher Mark Buehrle pitched a perfect game. In baseball history, starting in 1900 as far as most historians are concerned, there have been 263 no-hitters but only 18 perfect games (27 up-27 down). That's out of 779,118 starts which is .0023%!

That's pretty special and worth celebrating. I've been narrowing down the things I've been celebrating lately, trying to get the most quality out my everyday experiences.

My seemingly incoherent babbling has a purpose. Last week, we thought we had a pretty good handle on Charlotte's cancer. Her proton radiation treatments were over, we were all finally home and ready to begin the rest of the customized chemotherapy.

We got a call from the folks at MCV confirming an MRI appointment scheduled for early Wednesday morning and we just assumed it had been ordered by Dr. Khan or Dr. Tye since we had an appointment in the Nelson Clinic later that day. There we go assuming again.

So we headed off to the hospital and clinic that morning for what was her eighth MRI. After making it to the clinic, we were greeted with complete surprise by Dr. Khan when we told him about the MRI. "You had an MRI this morning?" He seemed confused but went to look at the scan just to see the results.

Here's where everything starts getting mucky. Dr. Khan came back in after a little while and said that after looking at this MRI and comparing it to the post 3rd surgery scan, he could see there had been changes. Here's your insight into the world of 'Dr. Speak' for these types of situations. When they say 'changes,' they don't usually mean changes for the good. He couldn't find the July MRI we did at MD Anderson, so he didn't have that one for comparison. Compared to the May MRI, parts of the cancer have grown. The thing is, it might be that the cancer grew more after the May MRI and the latest MRI might show that it has actually shrunk since then. If so, that's good and we can hope the updated chemo protocol will finish the job.

If the three MRIs show steady growth, even through the proton radiation treatment, that's very bad. The other thing is Dr. Khan only had a small amount of time to look at the scan and Dr. Tye wasn't even a part of the conversation, so there was very little information to be had which made us feel like we were being left in the dark. That's not the best state in which to leave our fertile, imaginative minds. The all-over-body-ache was back.

It certainly wasn't what we had hoped or expected. Did the super hi-tech proton radiation, the hottest thing in the world of cancer treatment, work at all? Was the time in Houston a gigantic waste? Did we do all that for no reason?

We felt so down for a bit that we didn't talk about it with anyone.

Here is where I tie it all together: a perfect baseball game won't change the world, but it is something that will be hard to match and, I think, worth remembering. I keep looking at Charlotte in those incredibly precious moments I get to spend with her and trying to devour everything about her. Every moment with her is a bonus that I cannot adequately describe in words and I want to remember these times.

Somewhere in all the mess, Rachel and I had one of THOSE conversations. It was in Chick-Fil-A with Charlotte sitting beside me eating her chicken strips dipped in barbeque sauce. We had both been stewing over the last conversation with Dr. Khan. We were thinking dark thoughts and going through worst-case scenarios in our heads. I think one can't help doing that sometimes and I do it all the time no matter how good things are going. I actually think it's one of the things that has helped me cope so well so far.

So there we were in Charlotte's favorite restaurant, speaking practically about 'what-ifs.' It was, by far, the most morbid but functional conversation we've ever had. Neither of us tends to shy away from difficult subjects and we both think it's wrong to not think about possible outcomes simply because it's hard to face. Denial has wreaked its own havoc on the world throughout history. I know, so has "the sky is falling!" mentality. Try not to worry. We're definitely not there yet.

In our various conversations lately, we've established that when Charlotte was first diagnosed, she was in the 80%+ survival rate category. When the cancer grew through the first couple rounds of chemo, we figure she dropped down to maybe 60%. If the scans show growth through the radiation, she reaches the 50%-or-less group. These are horrible things for a parent to have to think about but we wanted everyone to know where we are right now. We're not good. We've had some very difficult days since last Wednesday.

We have not given up hope. All this darkness is mostly because of what we DON'T know. That's where most fear comes from, right? Fear of the unknown?

We finally received the MD Anderson MRI from July and it seemed to be pretty inconclusive. Dr. Khan tried to temper the conversation by helping us understand that it can take up to eight weeks for the radiation to demonstrate its full effect on the brain. So we continued Charlotte's chemotherapy with a whole new set of drugs that had been recommended by the MD Anderson team. Fortunately, these drugs could all be dispensed either at home or through outpatient clinic visits. We resumed our activities, including physical and occupational therapy for Charlotte. Roger and I got back into *New Normal* work routine. Charlotte seemed to tolerate the new medications well. We approached those weeks with cautious optimism.

A few weeks before her next scheduled MRI (November 6), we noticed some tremors developing in her arms and legs and we were noticing more difficulty with motor skills. Because she was on so many medications, it was difficult to tell the source of the tremors. One of her medications actually had a side effect of Parkinsonian type symptoms such as tremors. She had begun to complain intermittently of headaches again. A dark cloud began to encroach on the sunny optimism to which we clung so desperately.

On November 6th, we sat in Dr. Tye's office; the very same treatment room where we had been on January 20th receiving the news of her initial diagnosis. As we sat there, gazing at the MRI scan on the computer screen, we faced the horrible reality we had feared. *Our options for treatment were gone.*

The tumor had continued to grow. Not only that, it was now placing pressure on her ventricles again, restricting the flow of her spinal fluid. This was the source of the headaches and tremors. Dr. Tye said that she would probably need surgery to install a shunt in her head to drain some of the fluid. This would be, at best, a temporary solution that would buy us time. Without it, she would probably be gone by Thanksgiving. With the shunt, we might have a few more months. *A few more months.*

We returned home that night trying to absorb the shock. I couldn't stop looking at Charlotte. I just kept thinking, "There is nothing left to do… but watch her die." I didn't want to miss a moment of any time we had left. Roger and I didn't really talk to anybody. We barely spoke to each other. It was too painful to talk. If it weren't for the fact that my daughter needed me to care for her, I would have crawled into a hole. I wanted to disappear. I wanted to push the reset button. I felt like I could face any reality except the one currently staring me in the face.

Less than 24 hours later, we found ourselves back in the hospital. While putting Charlotte to bed that night, she had a small but terrifying seizure. The entire event lasted less than 30 seconds but our survival instincts kicked into gear. Within minutes, we got her into the car and headed straight to the ER, calling her doctors along the way.

The seizure was a result of the growing pressure in her brain. Once she was stabilized, they admitted her once again to the seventh floor and we prepared for what would be her final surgery. Compared to the first three brain surgeries, this one was actually quite simple. A few days after her shunt surgery, we returned home from the hospital for the last time with a referral to Noah's Children, a local pediatric hospice team.

About a week later, the word *terminal* started floating around in my head. I thought of the obvious: my daughter has a *terminal illness*. On the other hand, there are many other definitions of the word terminal that gave new perspective to the situation:

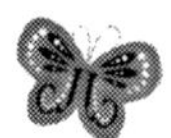

In grammar: That which cannot be further divided.

In botany: The flower growing at the end of a branch.

In engineering: An electrical junction where connections are made in order to redirect energy.

In travel: A port of arrival or departure; a place to say goodbye and a place to say hello.

We were sad beyond belief. Our hearts were broken. Yet I couldn't help but think of this as just the next part of the journey. I would happily trade in my tickets for another destination, but that didn't seem to be an option at this point.

We headed for the terminal. *The Network* was right there waiting for us at the gate.

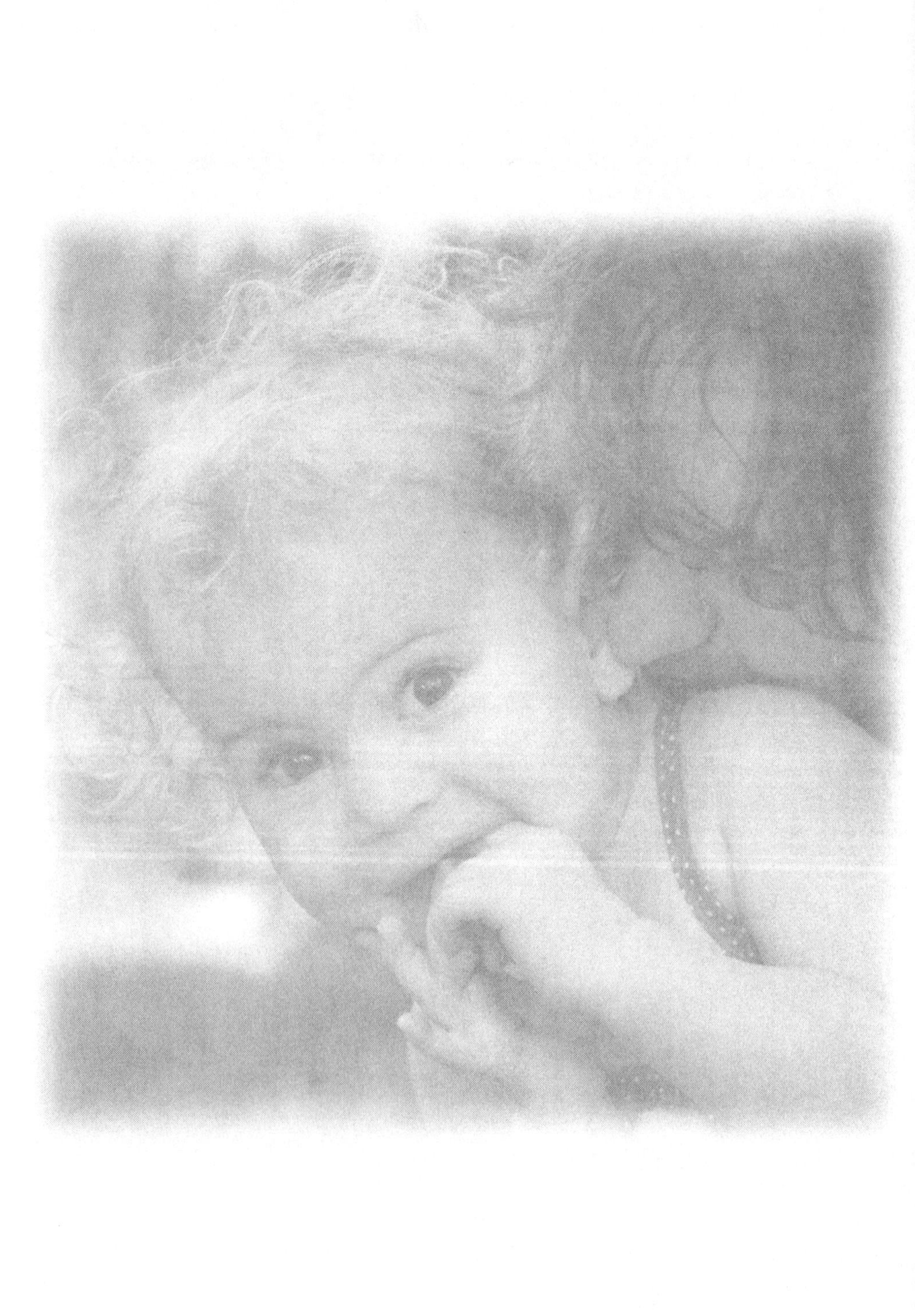

14— Charlotte's Farewell Tour

"Everything is on its way to somewhere."
—George Malley in the movie Phenomenon

I'm not sure how Charlotte ended up as such a girly-girl. I never fully embraced all things feminine when growing up. I liked dresses and makeup and a splash of pink here and there, but fashion and delicate femininity were not things that defined me. When Charlotte was born, her room was decorated in a neutral yellow with a Winnie-The-Pooh motif. We didn't find out our baby's gender ahead of time so we planned for all contingencies. Even after she was born, we didn't encourage the pink, although the closet soon filled with more dresses, pink onesies, and adorable hair barrettes than we could handle.

By the age of three, Charlotte was a bona fide fan of the princesses. She knew every single princess by name. She could sing the lines from many of the songs in *The Little Mermaid,* her favorite princess. She wore skirts and frilly dresses at every opportunity. Her favorite colors, as she loved to tell you, were "pink and purple."

Almost as soon as we got home from that last MRI, I called the Make-A-Wish Foundation. Earlier in the year, Charlotte had already selected her wish. She wanted to go "where the princesses are," aka Disney World. During the past year, she had also become enthralled with Tinkerbell and all of the other Fairies. Over 75 percent of Make-A-Wish requests are for Disney World-- so it's a popular destination. Charlotte had met with the Make-A-Wish volunteers while we were on the original protocol. At the time, we said that we hoped to take our wish trip in early 2010, after her scheduled treatments had been completed. So much for best-laid plans.

When I called the local chapter and explained the situation, they were extremely accommodating and called back within 24 hours to let me know that all we needed to do was pick a date after December 1st. Wish trips are usually one week in length; however, given the fact that so many of our family and friends lived in Florida, we wanted to make the most of the time we had left. With a little negotiation and a lot of prodding, I talked the director into granting us an exception. We would spend the first week of our trip at Disney World. This would be the Make-A-Wish experience. Then we would return the rental car and (at our own expense) finish the second week of our trip at my mother's house in Daytona Beach before going home.

Thus, our plans began for *Charlotte's Farewell Tour*. The first and most painful part of the process was getting a Do Not Resuscitate (DNR) order signed for Charlotte. Knowing that her condition was terminal, we needed to have this official document in place in case sometime during our travels we found ourselves needing to work with an unfamiliar team of doctors in an emergency situation. It is challenging enough that we sometimes find ourselves making decisions like these for our parents but it is something no parent should ever have to decide for their child. I remember going to the pediatrician's office to pick up the signed document. Usually a task left to the receptionists or nurses to relay, the doctor personally delivered the document into our hands, embraced us solemnly, and with tears in his eyes said, "I'm so sorry."

After the shunt was inserted into her brain, the tremors did stop somewhat. She was now, however, on doses of steroids and an anti-epileptic medication to keep swelling and seizures at bay. The steroids caused swelling everywhere (plus it stimulated her appetite). It became more and more difficult for her to walk without assistance so we got a larger stroller that would function almost like a wheelchair.

Roger and I didn't really go back to work for the rest of the year. We continued to keep up with the business from a distance, but we wanted to make the most of whatever time was left with her. Since we had started running our own business, our vacations had been limited to about two one-week breaks in as many years. So it was quite the shift in our lifestyle to suddenly not go to work every day. Our priority and responsibility was Charlotte: her comfort and her happiness. Everything else could wait. Nobody questioned our decision.

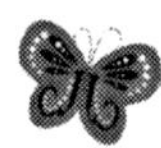

Our calendar soon filled with fun, once-in-a-lifetime activities for our family. Very little was off-limits. Charlotte could eat whatever she wanted whenever she wanted it. She could watch any movie she wanted. She could stay up all night reading books if she desired. We couldn't spoil her enough. As parents we had spent the first four years documenting so many "firsts": Her first words, her major physical milestones, her first movie in the theater, her first vacations with family. Now our life revolved around documenting the "lasts." Too many times, the "first" was also the "last."

We wanted Charlotte to have an opportunity to ride a horse. A shout out to *The Network* gave us two great riding events, including a group called Wings of Hope that actually brought the horses to our house and let her ride in our cul-de-sac.

One of our friends bore a strong resemblance to Mary Poppins. In fact, she had been Mary Poppins for a musical number in the Ashland Variety Show that year. Earlier in the year, she had visited Charlotte for a small tea party. We had even written a letter to Mary Poppins, ripped it up, and put it in the fireplace (just like in the movie). Mary, in full costume and accent, brought the letter with her (taped back together, of course) and they had a fabulous tea party complete with real china, scones, and jam! Mary Poppins was a constant feature in our house and frequently visited in Charlotte's final days.

About a week after coming home from the hospital, we were invited by another friend-of-a-friend to the Smithsonian in Washington, DC for a special treat. We received a private tour of the Natural History museum, including a "backstage" tour of their butterfly exhibit. The next day, we went to the National Zoo where we got our own private, up-close and personal meeting with Tai Shan the panda. Tai Shan and Charlotte were born on the same day (July 9, 2005). We had always thought it was cute that they shared the same birthday and figured that one day, someday, we would get up to the Washington area to see him. We not only got to see the panda, but we were also able to get closer than just about anyone. The trainer took us into a back area of the panda exhibit before the zoo officially opened. Charlotte and Tai Shan were inches from one another (separated by the cage, of course). It was amazing!

The week before Thanksgiving, a childhood friend of mine donated an all-expense-paid trip to Baltimore that included a night at a beautiful hotel in Inner Harbor, tickets to the Baltimore Aquarium, and five tickets to the Ravens/Steelers football game, including tailgating passes. We invited

Charlotte's babysitter Devon and her brother Patrick, both die-hard Steelers fans, and it was an amazing experience. Our seats were on the 30-yard line and about 20 rows back from the field. While we were amazed to have this incredible experience at an NFL football game broadcast on live television, I think most of the spectators within view of our seats marveled at this adorable little four-year-old in pink and purple, sitting the middle of the stands with these often gruff and aggressive-looking football fans. It was definitely a juxtaposition of images.

We returned from our Baltimore adventure to a spa day for the whole family sponsored by a local beauty salon. They treated all three of us to lunch. Charlotte got to have her nails, fingers *and* toes, painted. Roger and I each got a massage and I got my hair done.

Then it was off to Florida and Disney World. The trip was a once-in-a-lifetime experience. We stayed at Give Kids the World Village, which is a resort designed just for *wish families*. Each family gets their own, wheelchair accessible, two-bedroom villa. The village provided our meals and was an adventure park all on its own with features like a carousel, mini golf course, evening entertainment, and a playground designed after the Candy Land game. Each day, Charlotte received special gifts from the Village including picture frames, videos, and stuffed animals. There were opportunities to get pictures with Disney and Universal Studios characters as well as two pools, a spa for the kids, and horseback riding. There were 10 volunteers for every staff person at the Village and we were treated like royalty everywhere we went. You could get ice cream for breakfast, lunch, or dinner. As an organization that caters to families who have endured endless medical treatments and large amounts of stress, they knew just how to make us feel pampered, relaxed, and carefree. For just a little while, we could almost forget the reason why we were on vacation in the first place.

We spent three days at Disney World and one day at Sea World. During that time, we were joined by friends and family. They followed us to the park or met up with us in town. We even had our own photographer for part of the trip! One of our friends was a professional photographer and she volunteered her time to chronicle part of our trip. Thanks again to *The Network,* she traveled with us to Disney World for a few days. We were so grateful to have someone capturing those cherished memories.

As wish recipients, we got priority seating at shows and front row status on most of the lines. We would go to places where the lines stated 45-60 minute waits and we would get on the ride in about 10 minutes. Both Roger and I had lived in Florida for years, so this wasn't our first trip to Disney World. We didn't feel a huge need to see the whole park. This was Charlotte's trip. To that end, we spent the vast majority of our time in Fantasyland, riding the more easygoing amusements and finding characters to visit. Every time we saw a character, they would visit with Charlotte and us, never rushing our experience and always making us feel special. I will never forget the hug that Mickey Mouse gave us. He couldn't talk, of course, but he took one look at Charlotte and you could tell from the strength of his hug that Mickey "knew." He empathized and wanted us to know that he was thinking of us.

Sometimes Disney employees even sought us out. We were approached by more than one employee who would see us and say, "Follow me." They would then take us to an area where character visits or some other special event was happening. They wanted to make sure we wouldn't miss a thing. Thanks to them, we had a wonderful experience!

Because our wish trip came together at the last minute, we were unsure whether we would be able to participate in any of the frequently-sold-out Disney events like the character meals. Thanks again to *The Network*, we were given tickets to the coveted Princess Lunch at the castle. Charlotte got to meet every single princess and before lunch ended, her face was covered in lipstick kisses of every shade of pink and red!

The absolute highlight of the Disney experience was our visit with Tinkerbell and her fairy friends. Again, the wait to visit with these characters was supposed to be about 45-60 minutes, but our wish status bumped us up. We only waited about 10 minutes for the exciting event. The second Charlotte entered the room to meet Tinkerbell, Silvermist, and Rosetta, you could tell that she was enchanted. The room was made to look just like Tinkerbell's natural world with oversized flowers, friendly bugs, and a beautiful waterfall. Charlotte wasn't very steady on her feet, but she practically leapt out of Roger's arms to visit with the characters. You could just see the happiness on her face as she talked with each fairy. In the movies, each fairy is distinguished by having a special talent. There are water fairies, woodland animal fairies, flower fairies, and tinker fairies, fairies that invent tools or improve objects. The ladies discussed their talents *and* Charlotte's talents. The fairies decided, rightly so, that Charlotte was multi-talented. They gave hugs and kisses. It was magical in every sense of the word. I was so overwhelmed by the experience that I neglected my job as family videographer and forgot to record the entire scene as it happened.

The next day, we returned to the Magic Kingdom with my cousin and her young daughter, pretty much following the same route from the day before. When we got to the fairies, the girl who played Rosetta was the same one who had been there the day before. We think Tinkerbell was the same, but Silvermist was definitely a different person. This time, I readied myself with the Flip camera, hoping to catch something even minutely close to the experience of the previous day. When Charlotte entered the room, without any prompting from anyone, Rosetta exclaimed, "Charlotte! You came back!" They remembered her name! Then Rosetta proceeded to *remind* the other fairies about Charlotte: "Remember when she came to visit yesterday and we talked about her talents?" wink, wink. The other fairies got the drift and all chimed in to talk with Charlotte again. I don't know if Charlotte had ever been happier. It was definitely my favorite memory from that vacation.

People often ask us if we ever told Charlotte that she was dying or if we tried to explain what was happening to her. With all the frequent hospitalizations, Charlotte knew that she was sick. She also knew that all of the surgeries and treatments were things that "would make her head feel better." When her condition was finally deemed terminal, we struggled in finding the right words to explain this to Charlotte.

We had met with the doctors and the hospice team and they had shared the typical progression of the disease. Unlike some types of cancer, the progression of the tumor in her head should cause very little pain. As the tumor overtook her brain and spinal cord, her body would slowly begin to shut down. She would sleep more frequently. Eventually, she would stop eating and drinking. She would probably go to sleep and slip into a coma from which she would not wake.

How would you explain all of this to a very smart four-year-old whose only experience with death was the demise of a family goldfish, which we explained by telling her that Big Bird, the goldfish in question, "went back to the pet store"? After discussing the dilemma with our social workers and counselors, we decided that the best approach was to trust the process, knowing that the words would be there when and if we needed to explain the concept of death to our own daughter.

During that second day at Disney World, Roger formed the butterfly analogy. We were at the Winnie the Pooh playground. Charlotte's two-year-

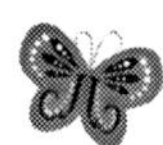

old cousin, Tricia, was running around with the other kids and Charlotte was sitting in her stroller with Roger by her side. She seemed somewhat frustrated by the fact that she couldn't play with the other kids. She had reached a point, as well, where sometimes she had a difficult time explaining what she wanted and this, too, frustrated her. Charlotte could still talk, but the words came out slowly. Sometimes she seemed to know what she wanted to say but stammered on the words or got "stuck" searching for the exact thing she wanted to say. This was challenging for a child for whom speech had been easy from an early age.

Roger started the conversation by reminding her about how a caterpillar turns into a butterfly. She had learned all about this in preschool, so she was familiar with the analogy. Roger told her that she was a caterpillar getting ready to go into her chrysalis. As the chrysalis grew around her body, it would become more and more difficult for her to move. Soon she would go to sleep and when she woke up, she would be a beautiful butterfly. The analogy worked in so many ways because as the steroids swelled her tiny body, she looked as though a cocoon really was consuming her. Charlotte understood this analogy and it carried us through until her death. Every time she would get tired or frustrated, we would remind her that she was working on becoming a butterfly. Becoming a butterfly was difficult work!

This analogy also helped when we needed to explain the process to Charlotte's friends. At the urging of our social worker, we held two events for children and their families to help the parents explain Charlotte's death to the kids. Many of the kids had already asked questions about her illness and it was going to be necessary to explain to them what was happening to Charlotte, as well as why they wouldn't see her anymore. We used the butterfly analogy and with the help of some volunteer grief counselors, we held an event we titled *Butterfly Away* where Eric Carle's *Very Hungry Caterpillar* was read. The counselors explained to the children that Charlotte would be like the butterfly. She would fly away when she died and the kids probably would not be able to see her anymore. Then the children and adults made their own butterflies, either to give to Charlotte or to keep as a reminder of her passing.

Around this time, we contacted a friend with graphic design expertise about creating a "CJ" butterfly that we could use on our website as a secondary symbol for the foundation that we were developing in her honor and as a memorial symbol for Charlotte. When we asked Madison to think of a design, we gave direction to make it pink and purple and to somehow reflect Charlotte. The CJ butterfly logo was born! Thanks to our graphic artist and our webmaster, the CJ butterfly was placed on our website the day that Charlotte passed away. It was animated to "fly" around the website in a seemingly random pattern.

The trip to Sea World was all about Charlotte's favorite birds: penguins. Charlotte always said they were her favorite "because they waddle but don't fly." She even had latched on to an adorable penguin puppet that she named Pinguino, the Spanish name for penguin. Another friend in *The Network* who lived in the Orlando area arranged to meet us at Sea World and help us get a backstage tour of the penguin encounter. During that day, we saw dolphins, sea lions, beluga whales, and polar bears, but the absolute highlight of the trip was the penguins. We not only got to see a King Penguin "up close and personal," but Charlotte got to pet him. He was almost as tall as she was!

As the first week ended, I was extremely grateful that we had one more week of "vacation." The trips to the theme parks were exhausting, so we almost needed a vacation from the vacation. After returning the rental car, we drove the hour or so from Orlando to Daytona Beach, my hometown, in a vehicle we borrowed from one of my high school friends *(Thanks again, Network)*. Our accommodations were a condo unit owned by my godmother. The three-bedroom place was right on the ocean and it was paradise! The weather wasn't very tropical (it was December after all), but we didn't care. Every morning we woke up to the sound of the ocean. We had views of the ocean from our bedrooms. One day, Charlotte just sat on the balcony watching the waves and eating cereal. All day. We kept asking her if she wanted to come inside, but she refused. I often remember that day and wonder what she thought about as she looked out on the ocean. Did she know that she was going to die? Was she happy? Did she know how much we loved her and how short her life would be?

Our second week was full of visits from friends and family but it was very relaxing in comparison to the first half of the trip. My mom organized two open-house events at the condo where friends and acquaintances could come and read to Charlotte. In a way, this was a warm-up to the reading vigil that was to come when we returned from Florida. We saw old friends and also met many who had been following our journey this year but had never met Charlotte before. The week culminated in a dinner with most of my extended family.

Although Roger and I put on a good face for the friends and family we encountered during the trip, I struggled with trying to enjoy the vacation

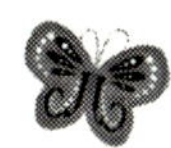

while worrying about Charlotte. Every day, I saw the clock ticking. I wondered how long we could continue to have *good* days. Would our trip be cut short? Would we find ourselves in the emergency room down here in Florida? Would she make it home?

One night, my father-in-law agreed to watch Charlotte in the condo while Roger and I took a moonlit walk on the beach. The weather was seasonably cool and incredibly windy and we soon migrated off the beach in search of some shelter. We found ourselves in a Denny's, one of the only restaurants open at 9:00 p.m., and we had another one of *those* talks.

"She's going to die. I have to say it out loud. Does it seem real?" I said to Roger.

"Not really," he replied. "I mean, it's real. We know it's real. It's still difficult to hear."

"Do you think she's happy?" I asked. "Do you think we're doing the right thing?"

"Of course we are! You saw her at Disney World. She's still laughing. She's still aware of everything that's going on," Roger said. "We just have to keep going one day at a time."

"There's a part of me that doesn't want to go home. There's this totally irrational part of me that thinks if we just stay here, she won't die. Does that sound crazy?"

"Not crazy at all," Roger agreed. "I'm right there with you."

"I still can't believe how OK I am with all of this. I mean, I'm *not* OK. Not by a long shot. I just think I've accepted it somehow. I think that's wrong."

"Rachel, it's not wrong. I think the fact that you've accepted the inevitable just means that you're ready for the next step. I think by accepting this we're able to be completely *with* her instead of looking everywhere for something that's going to cure her." Then he looked at me very solemnly. "We're going to be OK. Somehow. I'm not sure how, but I know we're going to be OK."

Then I started to cry. Like most of the times I cry these days, it's not a sob. It's just kind of a leak. The tears well up in my eyes and drip down my face. I am powerless to stop them. "This all just *sucks!* Do you know that? It *really, really, really* sucks!"

"Yeah," Roger says quietly. "I know." We held hands as we walked back to the condo. I felt safe just knowing that we were tackling this together.

The last day before we flew home, we saw noticeable change in Charlotte's physical situation. Roger and I saw some gradual changes that could have been attributed to many things, but the biggest shifts were in her balance and her sleep cycle. She was unable to walk, even with assistance, and she started sleeping for long periods of time. These were the signals the doctors had shared before our trip. We spent our last night in Florida at my mom's house (rather than at the condo) and my mom kept vigil by her side the entire night.

Many of the farewells during those two weeks were difficult. Everyone knew that this would be the last time they would see Charlotte. This was their chance to say goodbye. What do you say? What do you do? The farewell at the airport with my mom was probably the most difficult thing I'd ever done.

We made it home without incident, although we could tell that Charlotte was quickly fading. I had called the nurse at Noah's Children to let her know how things had changed as we prepared to come home. The nurse and social worker met with us the next day and assessed her situation. They definitely saw changes and proceeded to make updates to her medications. We came home from Florida on December 14th. Within three weeks, she would be gone.

The days that followed were powerful and surreal. Although we wanted to keep vigil over her, we knew that this could soon drain us physically and emotionally, especially when we didn't know exactly how long the process could last. We knew that our friends would want their chance to say goodbye to Charlotte but we didn't necessarily want a barrage of visitors to the house at all hours. We also knew that one of Charlotte's favorite things in the world was to read… and to be read to. From an early age, she soaked up language. She devoured it. As soon as she was old enough, she would "read" books to herself and could sit for hours and stay entertained. Some kids fell asleep with their bed full of stuffed animals. Charlotte would fall asleep surrounded by books.

In this spirit, we launched the reading vigil. We opened up our calendar and from 6:00 a.m.-10:00 p.m. on any given day, friends and family could come by to visit. If there were periods that we didn't want visitors, we blocked off the time. While the primary purpose of the visit was reading, friends were invited to sing, talk, and share in any way they desired. We put our webmasters to work on this project and they got an online calendar up and running before we returned home from Florida. This helped us create a schedule so that the house wasn't overwhelmed with visitors at any particular time.

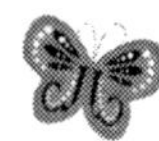

The reading vigil launched two days after our return from Florida. For the next two weeks there was almost a constant flow of visitors in the house. People read stories and sang songs. Most days, we were booked from 6:00 a.m.-10:00 p.m. with visitors staying anywhere from one to three hours. Mary Poppins came back for frequent visits. Charlotte's preschool class came and sang Christmas carols. Local musician and self-appointed Reynolds Family Fan Club President Susan Greenbaum came by with her guitar at least twice. In between visits from the nurses, the doctor, the chaplain, our pastor, and the social worker, the house was filled with a positive spirit. We even had family and friends from far away use Skype to read stories.

During the first week or so, Charlotte was alert and awake for many of the visits. Even when she slept, we encouraged people to read. Every time we asked her, she responded that she was enjoying the stories. We heard old favorites like Dr. Seuss and the *Give a Mouse a Cookie* series of books. We also heard new stories. People even told stories in foreign languages. *Green Eggs and Ham* was read in Latin! A friend of Roger's living in Amsterdam contacted us using Skype and read in Dutch. Another friend read stories in Italian.

I'm not really sure where Charlotte's fascination with Frosty the Snowman came from. When she was three, we would ask her what her favorite song was and one day she said "Frosty the Snowman." By her third Christmas, she had practically memorized the song. One of my favorite videos of Charlotte is of her singing at our employee Christmas party, about six weeks before her diagnosis. Someone had brought a karaoke machine and while nobody else wanted to embarrass themselves by breaking out in song, Charlotte had no problem standing up with a microphone in her hand, belting out "Frosty" while adding her own choreography to the mix. Even after the Christmas season had passed and the weather turned to balmy temperatures, Charlotte continued to tell anyone who would listen that her favorite song was "Frosty the Snowman." Anyone on her medical team knew this for a fact. This was especially humorous during our trip to Houston, Texas. In the middle of triple-digit temperatures and 99% humidity, you could find the nurses and physicians at the proton therapy center belting out "Frosty the Snowman" whenever Charlotte requested it. They even printed the lyrics and had them stored with her file so that anyone working on her team would be able to sing along!

Of course, once *The Network* learned of her fascination with Frosty, our home was filled with Frosty-themed gifts. We received blankets, dolls, and more copies of the movie than I ever could have imagined. Our favorite Frosty came from the Build-A-Bear workshop. Coincidentally, they were featuring a Frosty doll that year and one of Charlotte's Christmas gifts included a trip to create her own unique Frosty. Once the basic doll was created, she had to choose an outfit. We left the entire decision up to Charlotte and she, in turn, chose black jeans, black and white sneakers, a Harley-Davidson t-shirt, and a corresponding leather jacket. Someone jokingly referred to him as "Frosty the Bad Ass" and the nickname stuck. Even Charlotte referred to him that way. As we carried the Frosty from place to place, people would ask about him.

"Charlotte, is that Frosty?" someone might ask. She'd look up at the inquisitor with her adorable brown eyes and reply, "No, it's Frosty the Bad Ass!"

Living in Virginia, we are used to weather that pretty much follows the seasons; however, we are usually spared harsh winters. It can get pretty cold in Central Virginia but significant snow accumulations are the exception rather than the rule. Right after we returned from Florida, we got a huge storm that brought almost 14 inches of snow to the Richmond area. In honor of Charlotte's favorite song, people from all over the area (including many others who got snow all around the country) made snowmen for Charlotte and sent us pictures. Friends came over to our house and had their three boys build a snowman right outside her window. He was *huge*! We called him Frosty the Hutt. We received pictures of tall snowmen, short snowmen, pink snowmen, fairy snowmen, cheese ball snowmen, Blues Brothers snowmen, and of course, your garden-variety Frosties.

Christmas came and went. Charlotte hung on. New Year's came and went. She was still there. Right around the end of December, we thought she was slowing down. Her nutritional intake was practically zero. Although she was sometimes awake, she rarely opened her eyes and only occasionally responded with a nod or gesture that she had heard us speaking to her. Every time the doctor saw her, he would say, "Any day now." I called the nurse out in the middle of the night on at least three occasions thinking, *This is it*, only to find it was a false alarm.

Finally, on January 7th, right around noon, Charlotte's breathing pattern halted. It had been slowing down all morning. I would try to follow her pattern and find myself almost hyperventilating or passing out. Finally, she took a breath. Two minutes later she took another breath. And that was it.

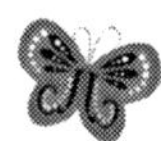

She wasn't in any pain. Her passing was calm and peaceful and beautiful. We had said our goodbyes. We had let her go. We let our butterfly fly away.

There were more than a few interesting anecdotes revolving around butterflies the day or two after her death. We received reports from at least three people who, in the cold winter, reported seeing butterflies outside the day that she died. We also heard stories of children (some of whom knew Charlotte, others who didn't) who, in the hours after her death, were pretending to fly around their house with butterfly wings or were talking about butterflies. Many of the parents who recalled these stories didn't even know that she had passed until after these events took place.

We had already decided to have Charlotte cremated. The funeral home came to claim the body and Roger carried her out to the receiving car. We went later that day to the funeral home to sign the necessary paperwork. We set about planning her memorial service… a final goodbye for our only daughter, our only child.

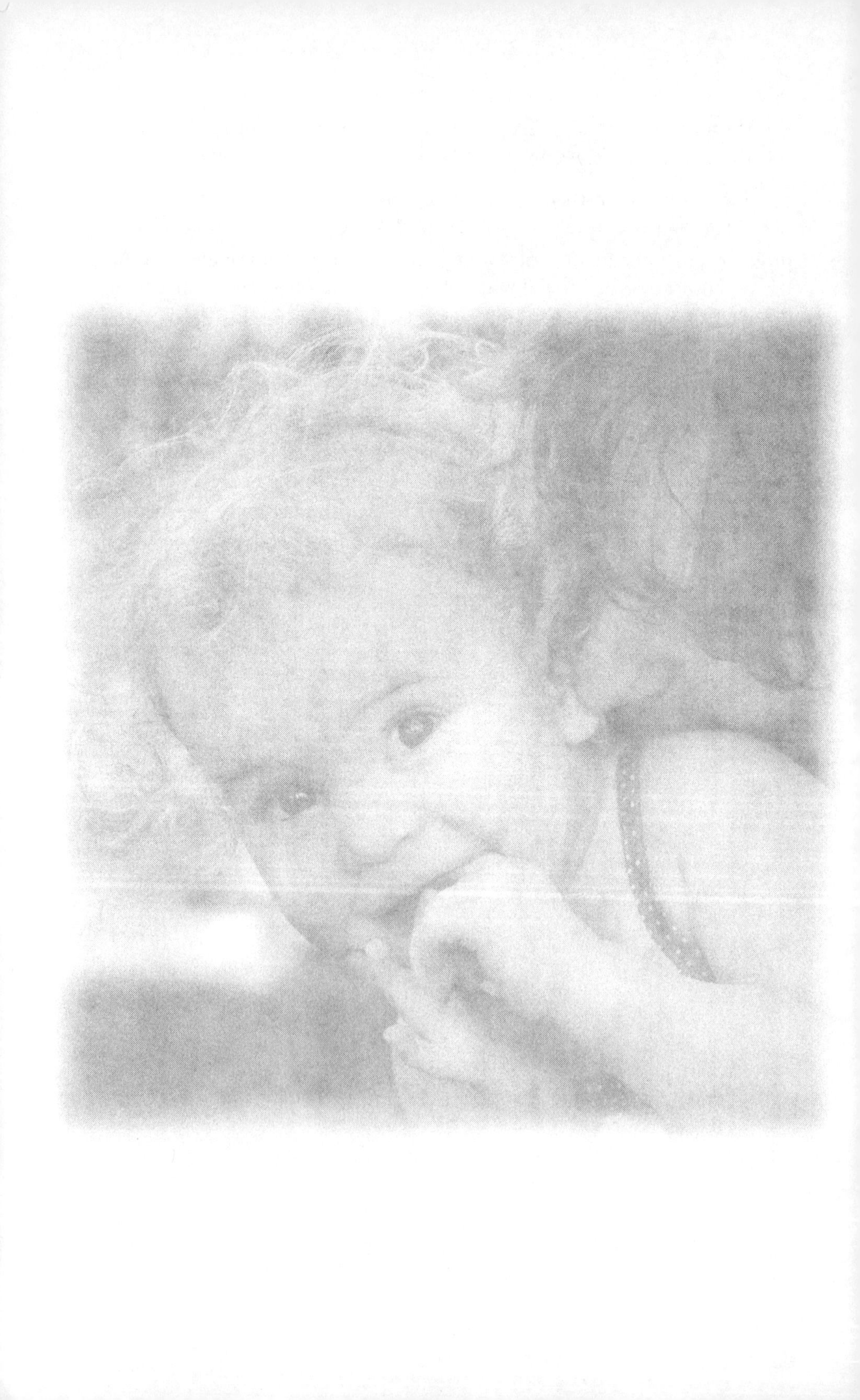

Charlotte Jennie was born on July 9, 2005 at 1:01 p.m. She weighed 6 lbs, 12 oz and was 20 inches long. These are the statistics that a mother never forgets. While my pregnancy was fairly uneventful, getting there was not an easy process. We didn't have the years of infertility troubles that some couples face, but I wasn't ovulating regularly and we sought the expertise of a fertility specialist. Some early attempts at facilitating conception with drugs (Clomid) or other methods were unsuccessful, but Roger and I didn't really consider in-vitro or other invasive and expensive treatments. Instead, we were investigating options for adoption. We had actually completed all but one class in a foster/adoption parenting training when we discovered, quite by chance, that we were pregnant.

Roger and I had talked about having more children and the tentative plan was to adopt any future children rather than having more biologically. We believed strongly in the concept of foster parenting and adoption, and had even talked about adopting an older child once Charlotte was also a bit older. We couldn't have her lose her "eldest child" status.

I thought of this often during the year of her *cancer*. We frequently heard the questions, "Is she your only child?" or "Do you have other children?" Yes. She was my only child. No. I have no other children.

I never was really sure how I felt about that. We certainly had enough to handle with our fledgling business and a child with full-time medical needs. I watched other families who dealt with frequent hospitalizations and the stress of treatment regimens. They struggled to balance their time with all of their children. They struggled to make sure *all* of their children received appropriate attention and care. We didn't have to try to explain to another sibling why Charlotte was dying. We didn't have to help our other children grieve. We could be alone in our own grief.

But when we lost Charlotte, we lost a huge part of who we were. Was I still a mother? Was Roger still a dad? She was our identity as parents and when she was gone, a bit of that identity was gone too. Of course, we would always be parents. She would always be our child. The reality, however, was stark.

Roger and I were both involved in online parent groups and in the weeks and months following her death, we sometimes felt awkward going back to participate in discussions. The groups had been incredibly supportive during the past year, but as we went back to engage in conversations about a variety of parenting topics, the conversation sometimes felt awkward. Would our comments be valid or even wanted now that we were childless? We did continue to participate in these groups on a limited basis, but we found that the scope of our participation narrowed significantly. I was more inclined to comment on an event going on in the area or a technical question about computer software, rather than parenting tips, potty training, or breastfeeding.

In the days after her death, it was bizarre to leave the house without checking to make sure she was OK. It was strange to look in the backseat of the car and realize we no longer needed a car seat there. After a year where life revolved around doctor visits, endless hospital schedules, and therapy appointments, it was alternately liberating and depressing to be able to just *go* anywhere we wanted (to the movies, on a trip, to dinner) without making childcare arrangements. It was like going around your house when the power is out. You turn a switch out of habit and then you are surprised when the light doesn't turn on. Then you remember: the electricity is not working. Damn.

I was surprised at how mundane activities really bothered me. Even before she died, I would go shopping and get frustrated. Walking the aisles, I would see things and realize, "I don't need that." Adorable dresses, toys, books, foods that she loved, there was no purpose. There were whole areas of department stores that were no longer applicable to my life. This continued even after her death and peaked with every national holiday.

Holidays were horrible. Every time one approached, I was flooded with memories of spending those days with Charlotte. I watched friends engage with their kids in Easter egg hunts, Fourth of July festivities, and all of the events surrounding Christmas and I was miserable. I was sad that we were trying to celebrate without her. During the first year following her death, social engagement was not my forte. I was jealous of friends who were enjoying the day while all I could think about was how much I missed her. I

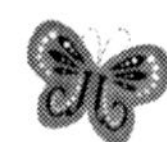

thought of all the memories that we had made in the past and all the future holidays in which Charlotte would not play a part. People would ask in casual conversation, "Did you have a good (name your holiday)?" and the truly honest answer was usually, "No. Not really."

Sometimes I just wandered through my day and wondered how the world kept going. I walked into public places and saw people laughing, talking, and concerning themselves with something that I thought was just *so* mundane. I wanted to scream at them and say, *"Don't you realize that my only child has cancer?"*

"Don't you realize that she is dying?"

"Don't you realize that my kid died today (yesterday) (last week) (last month)?"

I knew from a rational perspective that these strangers had done nothing to earn my ire, but I saw the world from a completely different frame of reference and it was frightening. I couldn't stand small talk. The perky, "How are you?" of the checkout cashier was enough to ruin my day. There was a part of me that really wanted to tell them the truth, and another part couldn't stand to ruin *their* day. That just wasn't right.

In fact, from the minute that her diagnosis was deemed terminal, we found ourselves frequently becoming the bearer of bad news. With everyone who had become a part of *The Network*, we sometimes found it odd that there were a few folks who knew us who still remained out of the loop on our current events. We would bump into people in the grocery store or at work who didn't know the latest. They would ask about Charlotte in the most benign, offhand way ("So, how's Charlotte these days?") and we would have to tell them the latest news. Usually it came as quite a shock.

As weeks and months went by, we found ourselves in social situations with strangers. *The Network* knew that Charlotte had died and knew that we were in the process of grieving, but we met new people at work and in other social situations who had never known our story. Obvious questions requisite to small talk would ensue: What do you do for a living? Where are you from? Do you have children?

How did we answer that question? In truth, the answer often was determined by the situation. My short answer was usually, "I had a daughter and she passed away in January." Of course, this would usually invite one of two reactions. Some people did not know what to say. There was an instant change in the tenor of the conversation. Either the topic would shift (as quickly as possible) or people would find themselves overcome with emotion. Sometimes the short answer gave us an opportunity to share our story. I usually didn't mind. I loved to talk about Charlotte! It was interesting to find ourselves in the position of comforting someone else. They would often say things like, "Oh, that's so sad," or "That's just horrible! The worst thing ever!" and all we could do was attempt a smile, nod politely, and agree. It really was the worst thing ever.

There were definitely situations where we side-stepped the issue completely. The answer to the question of children was usually, "Not right now." These were usually the "I'll never see this person again and it doesn't really matter" scenarios: the stranger giving me a pedicure, a waitress in a restaurant, or the cable repairman.

In my grief process, I found that my overwhelming emotion was jealousy. I was jealous of survivor families. Even when I could rationally tell myself that every survivor is one scan away from recurrence, I knew that I would trade that anxiety in a minute for more time with my daughter. I wasn't bitter towards these families. I didn't feel that they had something undeserved. I wasn't unhappy for them. I was just sad for myself. Four months after her death, I found myself wishing to be back in Houston or back in *any* hospital.

Why?

Life on *Hospital Time* was difficult, but it was always time with Charlotte. She was there. I could hold her and kiss her and watch another movie with her. I could hear her voice. I could read her a story. I couldn't do that anymore.

I was jealous of those whose lives had not been touched by cancer. I would hear parents complain about something trivial that their kids were doing or some dreaded thing that they *had* to do as part of that parental job description (changing diapers, putting a child in a time out, cleaning the house) and I would think about how I would gladly engage in those mundane parenting tasks that I myself used to dread. I was jealous of parents who celebrated all of those things that we were missing in our lives: the first day of school, vacations to new places, major milestones and triumphs. As a parent shared their joy, the scab on my heart was picked once again and the bleeding renewed. Sometimes I wondered whether I would ever be allowed to heal completely.

One of my first thoughts when her diagnosis was deemed terminal was all of the life events that she would never experience.

* She would never give a dance recital, take gymnastics, or play in the soccer league.

* She would never go to Kindergarten.

* She would never sing a solo in the Christmas play.

* She would never go to a slumber party.

* She would never audition for the school play or the marching band.

* She would never have a first crush…a first kiss…a first love.

* She would never take her driving test…and fail…and take the test again.

* She would never go to prom.

* She would never graduate from high school.

* She would never get married and have children of her own.

* She would never be the ambassador to China… or a famous actress… or a bean counter.

Most importantly, we would never get to see her participate in these experiences. When you greet your newborn child, you try to picture their life in one year, five years, fifteen years… through adulthood. You think of all the possibilities and while you can't prognosticate, you cherish every moment as it happens. You look forward to those opportunities and experience them right alongside your children. We had lost all of this and the reality was devastating.

I could ruminate on these things for hours to the point that it would almost make me sick. This concept of "what will never be" was the saddest part in the grieving process. Charlotte was amazingly smart and incredibly beautiful. What was the purpose in giving her only four years to share her life, her spirit, and her talents? At the same time, I thought of how she lived her life. She lived every day to the fullest. She didn't have time to nap. She didn't want to stop. She was always learning. She soaked up knowledge like a sponge and shared her charm with anyone who would allow it. Perhaps this was the important lesson for us to glean from this experience.

There are times that I wondered how I would feel if the course of her disease had gone differently. What if she had been diagnosed in January with an inoperable tumor? What if she had died on the operating table? What if she had come out of the surgery but had been seriously disabled with no hope of recovery? On the flip side, what if her course of treatment had dragged on longer and longer?

For Charlotte and for our family, the road was incredibly rough and the ending was incredibly sad, but I was grateful that the time that I had with her was great in quality even if it was not great in quantity. The best part is that I think we did all the right things. I'm proud of the parenting style with which Roger and I chose to raise our daughter. I cherish all the time I was able to spend with her. We had the best medical team possible that did everything in their power to fight that tumor. I have no regrets.

As to whether or not we will have more children, that is still a question for the future. Both Roger and I have very mixed feelings about that. Only time will tell if I can open my heart to another child and love them. There is pain and anxiety in that idea and right now it's too much to bear.

Every time I think about having another child, my thoughts seem to turn to our first pet, Mo. When we adopted Mo, he was a four-year-old beagle and he was the most perfect dog ever. He didn't bark. He was housetrained. He was a lazy dog that didn't require more attention than we could give. He wasn't the smartest dog on the block but he was sweet, adorable, and easy to care for. Mo was our first "baby" and he died of old age about a month after Charlotte was born. In the years that followed, we talked briefly about getting another dog. In fact, we had told Charlotte that once she "rang the bell" and ended her treatments, we were going to get a dog. Charlotte would watch the dog shows on TV and we would talk about which dogs she liked or didn't like. She had definite opinions. The simple fact of the matter is that we never got another dog because we were afraid that he or she wouldn't measure up to Mo. He was such a great dog and we were afraid that any other dog would pale in comparison to him. That's sometimes how I feel about having another child.

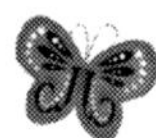

There is a large part of me that feels that parenthood began when Charlotte was born and it ended when she died. It is very difficult to explain but when I look at her life and our time with her, I see a sense of completion. It's not just the ending of a chapter but the ending of an entire book. I'm not sure what Volume 2 will bring. I'm not even sure that there will be a sequel.

As we prepared to say goodbye to Charlotte, we knew that *The Network* would play a key role in the process. We also knew that our church, wonderful as it was, would be too small a venue for her memorial service. We wanted the service to be a celebration of her life, not a mopey eulogy on her death. Thanks to our connections at Randolph-Macon College, we secured the use of the auditorium. Then we looked at the calendar and selected a date. Charlotte hadn't quite gone yet, but we knew her passing was inevitable within the next week and we wanted to give family and friends ample time to plan their arrival. Two friends volunteered to coordinate food and other necessary details and we set to work with our pastor to design the service.

> **Throw out the rule book when it comes to celebrating the life of your child. There are no hard and fast rules. Do what makes you comfortable and what feels right, not what you think you should do because of some so-called rules or conventions.**

It was beautiful and beyond anything I could have imagined. Our musician friends provided the music. It included some of our favorite (and her favorite) songs including "Wonderful World," "I'll Fly Away," and a sing-along finale of "Frosty the Snowman" and "Let's Go Fly a Kite." Our pastors from both Trinity and St. James the Less officiated and we even had a children's sermon. Roger and I spoke, sharing our favorite memories of Charlotte. As at our wedding, our siblings (Roger's sister and my brother) read scriptures. Everyone wore pink and purple at our request.

The auditorium could hold 600 people and it was standing room only. Our webmaster figured out how to stream the memorial service online for our out of town family and friends. At highest count, we had over 200 computer screens watching the service live and there was probably an average of 2-3 people at each computer terminal. Reruns of the service were streamed repeatedly in the days and weeks to follow. We had a videographer and two photographers capturing the day. After the service, everyone went outside and released pink and purple balloons on which we tied our messages to Charlotte. While it may have seemed overkill in the media department at the time, in the months to come, I was extremely grateful for all the people who captured these images. The time in the moment was a blur.

The days before her service had been cold and windy with threats of winter precipitation. It was January, after all. The day of her service, the weather was balmy, sunny, and clear.

There were so many people at the service that I only saw some later in the pictures. At the reception that followed, the entire hall was decorated with homemade butterflies that had been created by family, friends, and strangers in the week following her death. Many of the pieces were true works of art. Some had come from friends all across the country. The reception was full of donated food with some of Charlotte's favorites including macaroni and cheese, Chick-Fil-A nuggets, and a chocolate fountain. Charlotte's stuffed animals and dolls, many of which had been given in the past year by friends, lined the hall. There were musicians singing family-friendly songs. There was a craft and child care area for young kids, where they could make "worry doll" puppets from socks, butterfly bookmarks, and snowmen.

All of this came about because of volunteer efforts within *The Network*. Our friends, Kim and Meredith, took on the responsibility of chairing the event and the rest of the community contacted them with donations of time, food, artistry, and money.

It was a fitting tribute for a girl who was loved by so many in the community. We received notes afterwards from people saying that it was "the best funeral they had ever attended."

In the week that followed, the family that had flown in for the service returned home. Roger and I returned to work. My Aunt Phyllis stayed on for a few extra days to help put the house back together and organize some of Charlotte's things.

As our community helped us memorialize her life and process her death, many people sent cards or emails containing stories about Charlotte. Many of the stories were funny anecdotes. Some of our Romp n' Roll customers shared the first time they had ever met Charlotte and the impact that her life and her spirit had on them.

"I've continually thought back to a time in Open Gym in 2008. Charlotte had to tell me about the pets they had in her preschool class (gerbils). She spoke so amazingly well for a three-year-old! She then proceeded to pretend that she was a gerbil by placing the mats that form a circle [a large donut] *up on the side and getting in the middle as if she were in an exercise wheel. What great imagination and creativity! She then allowed E. to take turns with her in pretending to be a gerbil and even helped him out to show him what to do."*

"M. and I were visiting Romp n' Roll for one of the first times at Open Gym. We were the only ones there until a charming little curly-headed girl bounded into the room. She immediately introduced herself…not waiting for me to initiate. When I learned she was your daughter, I thought what a lucky little girl to have parents who own this awesome kids' gym. (The only thing cooler would be if you lived in a castle and owned a pony farm.) M. was just a baby so she wasn't able to do much in the gym. And Charlotte took it on herself, as the proud owner, to show us how to utilize each piece of equipment. The funniest part was that she used her impeccable charm and manners to ask my assistance in "spotting" her or giving her piggy-back rides. I can still clearly see her adorable smile and hear her angelic "please". And it worked. Almost to the point that I kept temporarily forgetting about baby M. just sitting over by the little rompers area. Through her exuberance, Charlotte was able to show me what fun being a toddler was! I wanted to take her home with us. I couldn't wait for M. to get to toddlerhood so we could laugh and play like sweet Charlotte did!

So it's a simple and brief moment in your child's life that I am recounting for you. But I am sharing it because I want you to realize what a lasting impression she made on me in that brief 30 minutes or so. I imagine that's how she lived her four years…to the very fullest when she could; charming people along the way. Charm is not always easy to find in other people's children. Cuteness and sweetness, yes. But charm is a sign of someone special. How fortunate you are to be Charming Charlotte's parents! And I know you realize that every day".

Yes, there was just something about her.

Charlotte had a spirit that was difficult to quantify. From the moment she was born, the nurses remarked on her beauty. Aesthetically, she was gorgeous. She had these blond curls that radiated like a halo and dark brown eyes that penetrated your soul. She had the sweetest voice I had ever heard. Physically, she probably most resembled me, but her spirit was a mix of daddy (free spirited and curious) and mommy (strong willed). She was a keen observer and smart as a whip. You showed her something a few times and she got it. Easily. At barely a year, she watched me screw the cap on a water bottle and then proceeded to do it herself. She talked at nine months and knew her ABCs before she was a year and half. She was reading before she was four years old. She was a social butterfly who wasn't shy about talking to others or finding out more about the world. We would go into stores and even as an infant she would say "Hi" to everyone. She never had a great deal of separation anxiety. She easily made friends and would talk to anyone who would listen.

When we went to the Smithsonian in November, we were waiting in the lobby for our host when a woman saw Charlotte and came up to say hello. We had never met or seen this person before, but she saw Charlotte from across the lobby and was clearly captivated. Charlotte was in her stroller so the woman asked Roger some questions. Was she sick? What was her story? Roger told her that she had cancer, a brain tumor. The woman asked if she was in treatment and Roger said, "Not anymore." When the woman asked what he meant, Roger explained that she had terminal cancer and had probably a month or so to live. The woman broke down and cried. She was clearly touched. We weren't really sure what to say or how to react but then the woman handed us a beaded bracelet. It still had the tags on it and I think she might have just bought it at the Smithsonian gift shop. She said, "Can I give this to her?" We graciously accepted her gift and the woman went on her way. She had that effect on complete strangers! It was crazy.

Yet with all of these stories, the phrase we heard over and over again was, "There are no words." It was impossible to try to explain the events of the last year (and yet here I am trying to do so in this book). Really, though, what I think that phrase meant was that it was not in words that we could find comfort. There was no rational explanation that we could find for why things happen or why the world was the way it was. And it was OK. We learned to be OK with not having all the answers. While there were no words, there was a spirit of grace and peace that transcended the entire experience. That was the spirit by which Charlotte lived her short but full life.

Epilogue: Charlotte's Legacy

"Do not judge the bereaved mother. She comes in many forms. She is breathing, but she is dying. She may look young, but inside she has become ancient. She smiles, but her heart sobs. She walks, she talks, she cooks, she cleans, she works, she IS, but she IS NOT, all at once… She is here, but part of her is elsewhere for eternity."
--Source Unknown

What does it mean to "get over it"? This term gets bandied about in support groups, grief circles, counseling sessions. I have seen parents get upset when they are asked years after the child's death, "When are you going to get over it?" What is "it"?

Grief is a process. I don't think you ever completely finish grieving the loss of a loved one. Most psychologists and grief counselors would tend to agree with me. You will always wish you had one more day, one more minute, one more opportunity to share the love. At the same time, you live with the hope that there will come a day when it doesn't hurt quite as much. There will be a day when you don't wake up with the ache in your heart every time you think of their smile. There is no set timeline. The process is different for everyone and it can often be affected by the death process itself.

Remember Kübler-Ross's five stages of grief? Although that theory has dominated the grief counseling world for decades, there are other schools of thought that propose grief without stages. In her book, *The Truth About Grief: The Myth of Its Five Stages and the New Science of Loss*, Ruth Davis Konigsberg proposes that grief is not as predictable and able to categorize as Kübler-Ross originally theorized. Discussing the idea in a magazine article in *The Christian Century*, author Thomas Long comments:

"Grief is not mainly a psychotherapeutic unfolding; it is a perilous, unruly, and emotionally fraught narrative task. When someone dies, the plot threads unravel, the narrative shatters, and those who are part of the story 'go to pieces.'

The work of grief is to gather the fragments, and to rewrite the narrative, this time minus a treasured presence."

This thought resonated with me. While I understood and acknowledged those feelings of anger, denial, sadness, and bargaining that Kübler-Ross used in her compartmentalized explanation of the grief process, this idea of rewriting the narrative of our lives made even more sense. With every loss, the process was different. The pieces were shattered in different ways. Sometimes the healing, or the repair, took on different forms depending on the way the damage was done.

In my early experiences with death, the loss came instantaneously. There was no warning. My father took his own life when I was eight. While I know, looking back, that there were warning signs, as an eight-year-old, I was clueless. One day my father was there and the next day he was out of my life. I actually didn't fully grieve his death until I was a teenager. Five years after he had died, I realized the anger and sadness that had built up inside of me. I wished for a different life. I mourned my existence in a single parent household with a mom who couldn't understand me (I was a teenager. Angst was abundant at the time.). Eventually I found a peace in my life and I accepted my father's death. I realized that the life I was living was rich and full and happy. I accepted that it was my father's selfish act that was the problem… and that he was the one who had really lost. At one point, I just came to the realization that I had lived more years without my father than with him and it was time to move on. There was a clean break at the seam, but the process of hemming the edges was a slow one. The repair took time but there came a point when the work was finished. There would always be signs of a tear but it was a repair that could be lived with.

Other early experiences with death were similar. My grandfathers died before I could really remember them and both of my grandmothers died suddenly in their sleep, one when I was nine and the other when I was twenty. There was no long-term illness, no battle with a raging disease, no endless hospitalizations. It was just a phone call. One day they were here and the next day, we were preparing for their funeral. Without a long, drawn-out process, my last memory of them was the last time I saw them alive. Fortunately for me, those were happy memories. The repair process happened faster in these situations. The hems were easier to hide within the stitching.

In the weeks following Charlotte's death, our grief process just continued along the path it had already started. Grieving actually began the day of her

 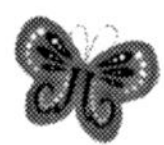

diagnosis. Our world was torn asunder. This was not a clean break but a messy shredding of the garment. Every time we reached a new milestone in her treatment process, every time an MRI gave us bad news, we faced more damage but we also worked simultaneously to repair the damage as much as we were able. We accepted her death long before she actually died. That didn't mean that we weren't still angry or sad after she was gone. We were angry. We were sad. We were jealous of others. The feelings fluctuated from day to day. We weren't, however, bitter or in denial. We didn't blame anyone. We didn't regret any choices we had made. Once we reached that acceptance stage, we could truly begin to heal. There was a part of us that reached acceptance even before her death.

After her passing, we realized how tired we were. Roger and I went away on a retreat for a few days immediately after her death but before the memorial service, and we slept. We rested and allowed our bodies to re-energize. Returning to work and finding a new routine (hey, there's that *New Normal* again) helped as well.

Our life shifted to *another* normal. We returned to work. We slowly began to interact with others socially, accepting invitations to parties, dinner events, and social occasions. We busied ourselves with the mundane and the spectacular. The missing piece was Charlotte. There was no daycare or school. There was no carpool or play dates. There were no bedtimes or bath times to schedule. Our lives were never the same again.

As the year went on, we were reminded of the milestones that had marked the previous year. The grief process started all over again. We cycled through depression, anger, denial, bargaining, and acceptance yet again. While we continued to live our lives, we experienced pain, jealousy, and true heartache in between serenity and peace. There was no rhyme or reason to the way we might feel on a particular day. Sometimes it would hit us in the strangest moments.

We thought in that year of the anniversary of her diagnosis (only four days after her memorial service), dates when she had surgeries, was admitted to the hospital for chemo, the day she lost her hair. We tried not to dwell on these dates but commemorate them in ways that were appropriate. I found myself looking at pictures of her and sometimes wondering if the whole year had not just been a bad dream. Was she real? Did this actually happen? The surreal nature of her brief existence and intensely final year on this planet somehow made it seem like something that had been imagined. The shredded narrative was slowly being repaired. It was a long and arduous process.

Roger found words early in the grieving process that resonated with him. Neither one of us can remember the source of the quote but it became kind of a mantra for us: *"Don't be afraid to look back but don't stare. It's OK to commemorate. Just don't dwell."*

One of the greatest compliments that we received from people after her death was when they told us how observing our experience and watching how we dealt with the tragedy of the past year had made them a better parent or a better person. People frequently mentioned that they cherished those experiences with their kids… even the mundane or trying ones… because they realized how precious life could be. They made a conscious effort to spend more quality time with their kids and their families. They began to reach out to others in need and looked for ways to help other families like ours. That was powerful. That was meaningful. At the very least, it helped me think that maybe there was some grand purpose for all of this tragedy.

We frequently heard that phrase: *Everything happens for a reason.* I have mixed feelings about that statement. In Michael J. Fox's memoir *Always Looking Up*, he quotes Michael Manganello. He is a stem cell advocate who worked closely with Christopher Reeve after his tragic accident. In response to people who cited Reeve's accident as fulfilling a higher purpose, Manganello is quoted saying, "No, this just sucks. It doesn't happen to anybody for a reason. Sometimes bad things happen, but it's how you deal with those things that matters." I don't think I could say it better myself.

Even before Charlotte's diagnosis was deemed terminal, we had talked about capturing the amazing force of *The Network* and turning it into something that could pay it forward and help others. We wanted to be able to help other families with the same kind of generosity that we had experienced. The day before her death, CJ's Thumbs Up Foundation (CJSTUF) became a certified corporation in the state of Virginia.

During her life, we alternated frequently between Charlotte and CJ. Roger liked the acronym the name created because CJ was one TUF little kid. She endured more medical procedures in her tiny life than Roger and I had experienced in our almost 80 combined years. The "thumbs-up" sign came from the day of her first surgery. When she was in recovery, Dr. Tye was trying to get her to respond to his questions. While it was difficult for her to talk, she was able to give us a thumbs-up for good and a thumbs-

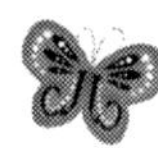

down for bad. The symbolism stuck. Two years later, the nation watched as Congresswoman Gabrielle Giffords recovered from brain surgery to repair the damage caused by a gunshot that attempted to claim her life. Rep. Giffords couldn't yet talk, but she gave a "thumbs-up" from her hospital bed as she attempted to communicate with her friends and family. I couldn't help but think of Charlotte.

The mission of CJ's Thumbs Up Foundation is to help families of children with chronic and life threatening illnesses with the kind of monetary support that *The Network* provided in our time of need. We don't fund research. We don't find a cure. We don't fix someone's financial crisis. We just make an unbearable situation a little more bearable.

As the organization grows, we hope to widen our geographic scope as well as give to more families each year. Thanks to tremendous local support and a large amount of money remaining from fundraisers that were held during Charlotte's illness, we gave away over $30,000 in our first two years, to over 40 families. While we may have lost our daughter, we are looking forward to investing our time and energy into an organization that will help others and allow the legacy of her spirit to live on.

In the years following Charlotte's death, our lives have changed in many ways. Roger and I relinquished ownership of Romp n' Roll in May, 2011. We had struggled to keep the business going but the economic climate continued to have other plans. Less than six months after Charlotte's passing, I sought a full-time job back in special education while Roger tried to continue with the business. It was a losing battle. Our time is now divided between work with the foundation and other professional endeavors. We continue to take life one day at a time, greeting the turn of each season with memories of the past and hope for the future.

9 781928 662259